Dedicated to all the sufferers of any mental health issue and their loved ones, and to those working tirelessly across all spectrums around the world to bring a better understanding and awareness of mental health issues through research, support and treatment.

> By openly talking about mental health, we can pull the trigger on mental illness.

Thank you for purchasing this book,
you are making an incredible difference

All of our **Pulling**the**trigger**® products have substantial
enterprising and philanthropic value which generate contributing
proceeds towards our global mental health charity,
The Shaw Mind Foundation

MISSION STATEMENT

'We aim to bring to an end the suffering and despair caused
by mental health issues. Our goal is to make help and support
available for every single person in society, from all walks of life.
We will never stop offering hope. These are our promises.'

Pulling the Trigger and The Shaw Mind Foundation

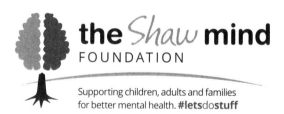

The Shaw Mind Foundation (www.shawmindfoundation.org) offers
unconditional support for all who are affected by mental health
issues. We are a global foundation that is not for profit. Our core
ethos is to help those with mental health issues and their families at
the point of need. We also continue to run and invest in mental health
treatment approaches in local communities around the globe, which
support those from the most vulnerable and socially deprived areas
of society. Please join us and help us make an incredible difference
to those who are suffering with mental health issues **#lets**do**stuff**.

CONTENTS

PART I ADAM'S STORY

PART II Pullingthe**trigger**®

INTRODUCTION

COURAGE NOT FIGHT

Accept Your Mind, Own It For What It Is.
This Takes Courage, Not Fight

All my life, from being a little boy to a fully grown man, I tried to suppress my thoughts and anxiety because I knew no better and because I felt compelled to fight them. I was frightened, ashamed of and appalled about my mind and my crippling thoughts. It was terrifying, lonely and debilitating. I constantly felt that I was on the edge of madness and that no one or nothing could help me. It felt like a war I was gradually losing every day as my strength would deplete and my energy drain. The day I brought Lauren into my life, some thirty years' later, was the day I stopped fighting and my life changed forever. The day I truly accepted my thoughts and truly embraced them was the day I began to take control; this made surviving my anxiety-based mental illness possible, but more importantly made my recovery inevitable. A new life was beginning for me. No words will ever be enough to thank my wife, Alissa, my beautiful children and, of course, my therapist and colleague Lauren Callaghan for all their unconditional love and support.

Adam Shaw

Adam Shaw: We can all change the game on mental health recovery. It's time for a new way of thinking, so let's make recovery possible for all.

Providing this service through our recovery approach and charity foundation is my passion. Pain and suffering through anxiety-based mental illness has played a big part in my life through childhood, adolescence and adulthood, and at times has come terrifyingly close to destroying me. However, I promise you that survival and recovery can and will happen, as we guide you through our method of **Pulling the Trigger (PTT)**: a combination of **Cognitive Behavioural Therapy (CBT) with a Compassion-Focused Approach**. I can assure all my fellow sufferers, families and loved ones of sufferers, and indeed anyone supporting the **PTT** movement, that through your support and contribution by purchasing this definitive and inspiring recovery approach, you will not only help ensure your own recovery, or that of your loved one, but just as importantly you will also be helping and supporting those most vulnerable in our society and those who are also trapped in a cycle of despair through mental health issues. We achieve this through our global charity organisation, The Shaw Mind Foundation (www.shawmindfoundation.org). It is our mission to show sufferers from all walks of life and around the globe that they are not alone because help and support is available and accessible. Sufferers and their loved ones don't have to give up hope because survival and recovery is more than possible. We promise this.

Within this recovery approach, Lauren and I want to give you the very best of our experience in dealing with Obsessive Compulsive Disorder (OCD), anxiety, panic attacks and related depression while we encourage, help and support you as you lay your torment to rest. And be assured that's exactly what you will do if you follow our journey. Our approach is a simple yet highly effective treatment for mild to severe anxiety-based mental health issues and is located in Part II of this book. The first section of this book contains my personal story; a journey through the severe struggles I have faced with mental health issues throughout my life. While my story is one primarily dominated by OCD, it is important to stipulate that it has relevance on so many levels to all those suffering with various anxiety-based mental health issues. I want sufferers and their loved ones to understand my story so they are able to identify the elements which also contribute to their own personal suffering. We have added my story to Part I of this book by way of an introduction to our **PTT** approach and while we encourage you to read and digest my story as a platform to begin your recovery, the magic within this book comes in Part II – the **PTT** approach which will help lead you to recovery and to a life free of OCD, anxiety, panic attacks and related depression.

I call it an approach. In fact, it's more of a survival and recovery manual. Let me explain. At the time of writing, I'm a businessman operating various companies in the legal services industry and living in Lincolnshire, UK. I have a wonderful wife, five great children and a warm and supportive extended family. One would say I have many of the trappings of success for which I consider myself a very lucky man. However, this has not always been the story of my life. There was a time when my mind seemed to be shattered into so many pieces that I felt I could not continue living. The OCD and extreme anxiety that I'd suffered from childhood had spun completely out of control, causing me panic attacks and many regular suicidal thoughts.

In the middle of my last major episode of anxiety and panic, which resulted in my contemplating suicide, I'd attended the Accident and Emergency (A&E) Department of my local hospital, desperately begging them for help. The UK's National Health Service (NHS) being what it is, the A&E Department simply didn't have the resources within its mental health service to do something for me there and then. I felt like I was going crazy and wished someone could put me into a deep sleep that would last a year or more. I just didn't want to exist any more through this acute mental torment I was suffering from.

When I stood on that bridge, staring at the train tracks below and wondering if I had the courage to jump, I was at my lowest ebb. 'If I can't beat this now,' I thought, 'I never will.' And this was from the man who had everything to live for, and many of the things other people may envy. This wasn't a cry for help; I was deadly serious about ending it all. I was in an extremely desperate state of mind, but equally I was rational in my thinking when it came to suicide.

I had ensured my estate was in order so my wife and children would have a secure future. Furthermore, I was deeply concerned for the driver of the train. I didn't want his or her world turned inside out by going through the horror of seeing someone jump in front of a high-speed train and be unable to do anything. My rationale to achieve this was to jump just as the first carriage passed under the bridge. Looking back, I guess I didn't take everything into consideration as the thought never even entered my head about the poor person who would discover my body.

I didn't jump that day. I was almost convinced it was the right thing to do. But something – a tiny bit of hope, perhaps – stopped me from going over the edge. After that day, I told myself that if I got better I would somehow help other people suffering from the anxiety and OCD which had crippled me. At that stage I realised that only by taking matters into my own hands would I start to recover. I make no criticism of the NHS in the UK; it provides an excellent service within its budget. But I needed help there and then, and luckily I was in a position to fund such assistance myself. I realise that many others aren't able to do this, which is why I made the vow to help my fellow sufferers and their families. This book and the recovery approach contained within it is the first step on that road to tackle an illness that affects many people across the world, and probably more alarmingly, the millions more who have yet to be diagnosed.

How did I get better? How did I get to the point in my life where I can now say I've recovered? Well, it's a long story but not a particularly complicated one. I was fortunate enough to meet Lauren, an industry-leading therapist and the co-author of this book and PTT approach, who introduced me to a completely new way of approaching my illness; how to accept the thoughts I was having, embrace them and by doing so, control them. The three short words which sum up these techniques are **Accept, Embrace** and **Control**. Three words that form the basis of everything Lauren and I will teach you in this recovery approach. There is nothing more to it than that.

- You must **accept** that you have anxiety and understand that it is your current state of mind. We do not fight or question our state of mind; we allow it to be.

- You face the fear, **embrace** it, openly letting your fears in and proactively moving towards them. You do not run away by distracting yourself or by trying to 'keep your mind occupied'.
- By doing these things, you eventually learn how to **control** your mental health to see it for what it is – a collection of thoughts; no more, no less. It's about understanding that sometimes control means letting go and accepting that it's OK not to be in control of your thoughts, sensations and initial emotions attached to them.

We have called this approach '**Pulling the Trigger**', or '**PTT**' for short. It is an approach that has evolved from the techniques which Lauren introduced me to, but it also derives from our combined experience, wisdom and expertise, which eventually became the **PTT** approach.

Pulling the Trigger is simple, and deliberately so. Not being a qualified medical specialist, I have no wish to confuse readers with a lot of theorising about anxiety and OCD. This, to me, is unhelpful, and I feel it can actually lead the sufferer down the wrong path, as it did to me over the years. I believe that my experience of suffering with severe OCD and extreme anxiety and finally recovering has led me to a place where I am in the strongest position possible to help my fellow sufferers. This book and the approach contained within it is therefore written, in part, by a long-term and severe OCD and extreme anxiety sufferer, and is aimed at fellow sufferers and their families.

That said, it is through bringing Lauren into my life, a leading anxiety-disorder specialist, that I was finally able to find the courage, mindset and support to break free from my suffering. Therefore, I want to give all my fellow sufferers the very best chance of recovering by having my experience, and the expertise of one of the most talented therapists in the industry, contained within this book, ensuring the reader has the techniques to survive and recover, but just as importantly to live a life with purpose post-recovery. It is a passion and an ethos of ours to show that through the PTT approach and the treatment we will introduce to the sufferer, these techniques and new ways of thinking can also be embraced in your future so you can recapture your zest for life. Why stop at recovery? Help and understanding in this area is so difficult to come across, as I discovered over the years; the information contained within our PTT approach will finally break down that barrier and give you the help, support and techniques for survival and recovery. It gave me the life beyond that I was frantically seeking for most of my life.

I do understand that for almost all of us suffering as I have done, the journey into acceptance can take quite a while. The instant panic and intense dread of an anxiety-based mental illness such as I had with OCD feels not only debilitating to the sufferer, but brings with it extreme isolation and loneliness when unwanted thoughts and anxiety kick in. For a long time we have been living with thoughts that have dominated our lives, told us to behave in certain ways and taught us that certain patterns of behaviour are the only ones which will help us avoid the anxiety and OCD that torments us. Ironically it is the very avoidance of anxiety and OCD, panic attacks and related depression which makes it feel twice as bad. I and millions of other sufferers have tied ourselves in knots trying to 'understand' what is happening to us, asking why it is that we have to suffer, doing everything we can to avoid bringing on another episode.

Do not get confused between fight and courage when it comes to recovery. Anxiety thrives on and feeds off your internal fight and struggle while you are trying to conquer this illness, but it runs scared of courage as you start to take the steps to face it and see it for what it is; a misfiring emotional response driven by fear and without substance.

Only by *accepting* and *embracing* anxiety and OCD will you ever learn to *control* it, and finally stop it plaguing your life and those of the people around you. Instead of running away from it, walk boldly towards it. Ask it to visit you, again and again. Stare it full in the face and tell it to do its very worst. Because if you do, do you know what will happen? It will back down, shrink away and slink off. Not immediately, but I absolutely promise you that in time, that is exactly what will happen. The technique of **Accept**, **Embrace**, **Control** will eventually allow your mind to desensitise itself to the obsessions and compulsions that swirl around it. Look at it like a parachute jump: at first, the fear you feel on exiting the plane is huge. Next time you do it, you'll be fearful again, but perhaps less so. Then you do it again and again, and eventually so often it becomes second nature. That's desensitisation. You walk along the high wire, you lean out of the basket of the hot air balloon, you swing across the circus tent on the trapeze, and each time you do it you become that bit more confident, and less fearful. That is how you tackle anxiety, OCD and depression, and the PTT approach will give you everything you need to finally rid your mind of the obsessions, compulsions and anxieties that dominate your thoughts and ruin your everyday life.

The best way to show you how to achieve all this is firstly to take you through my own story, chapter by chapter in Part I of this book. I'm not a doctor, or a therapist or any kind of medical specialist. I'm an ordinary man from the UK with a problem that millions around the world suffer from; worse still, the majority will suffer in silence, so I hope you will be able to relate to at least some of my story. As each chapter progresses in Part I, Lauren will add her thoughts and commentary to what I've been describing in my own life, and then in Part II of the book we will introduce our recovery approach – Pulling the Trigger. Within our PTT approach in this book, we have also included individual sections on support for anxiety and OCD sufferers from a family perspective, fitness and diet, and also our view on using medication for these problems.

I have achieved much in my life, despite my illness (and sometimes because of it – where there are negatives there are always positives!) but this is the biggest and, personally speaking, the most important project and journey I've ever embarked on. Only my therapist and my wife, Alissa, know the full story of what happened to me and how I recovered. I will be sharing deeply personal information with family, friends, colleagues, employees and you, the reader. It's not easy telling people that your illness has pushed you to the very limits of sanity but it's the truth, and I pride myself on my honesty. That's all I have, and I hope that my honesty helps you through your own troubles and serves as a secure platform for you into our PTT approach.

Finally, a word about the title and the approach we've devised of the same name. Many things have triggered my OCD and anxiety, but for an equal number of years I shied away from those triggers, hoping that by avoiding them the illness would go away. It didn't. Now I see that if I'd gone towards that trigger and just pulled the thing –

and I don't mean in a suicidal sense, but simply as a metaphor for facing fear – I would've sorted out my difficulties years ago. Through this book and approach, I want you to do the same. Good luck on the journey, and stay with it, even when it becomes tricky. Recovery is within your reach. We promise this.

Lauren Callaghan: Thank you for picking up the book and having the faith to read and follow our recovery approach. Firstly, a little about me. I'm originally from New Zealand where I studied both Law and Psychology at university. I was heading towards a career in law, and even completed my legal training and was admitted to the Bar, until I changed my mind and decided to continue my postgraduate studies and train as a clinical psychologist. I was interested in human behaviour, and I wanted to be in a profession that helped people and where you could see the direct impact of your hard work in making positive changes for individuals, families and communities. I eventually moved to the UK and worked at the renowned Centre for Anxiety Disorders and Trauma (CADAT) at the Maudsley Hospital in London. While there I also worked in the National Services Team for OCD and BDD (Body Dysmorphic Disorder), a UK government-funded programme to treat the most severe cases of OCD and BDD around the country. I then worked at the National Services CBT (Cognitive Behavioural Therapy) programme for severe and complex anxiety disorders at the Bethlem Hospital, part of the Maudsley Hospital group, which again was a national specialist unit in treating OCD and BDD. I appeared as a therapist on *BEDLAM*, a BAFTA-winning documentary on the treatment of severe OCD and I am a frequent guest speaker on BBC radio about OCD and anxiety problems.

In addition to my clinical psychology training, I am a very experienced and certified CBT therapist. I am a national-level specialist in OCD and BDD, and I teach and supervise psychologists and CBT therapists, as well as presenting at national and international-level conferences on these topics. I am a guest lecturer and honorary researcher at the Institute of Psychiatry, King's College, UCL, where I have both taught and evaluated the CBT training courses and where I am currently involved in research and evaluation of new OCD and CBT treatment methods.

I am passionate about giving back to the community and promoting evidence-based psychological treatments, and until recently I was the chair of the Communications Committee of the British Association for Behavioural and Cognitive Psychotherapies (BABCP). I am actively involved in supporting OCD and BDD charities in many ways, including promoting awareness of anxiety disorders and presenting at annual conferences for sufferers and their families, as well as raising awareness and the profiles of these illnesses by fundraising for the charities. Today, I run two private practices in London, which specialise in a number of disorders including anxiety and obsessional disorders, including OCD and BDD.

The PTT approach found in Part II of this book is an effective treatment for OCD, anxiety, panic attacks and related depression. You will often hear the words 'stress', 'worry', 'anxiety' and 'panic' in relation to everyday occurrences; 'I am stressed at work', 'I hate public speaking, I always panic', 'I worry about that all the time!', 'That makes me feel really anxious' and so on. These terms are often used interchangeably and for all types of situations. In fact, they are all referring to the same human experience, although this human experience may vary in severity and duration. For the sake of clarity, we will use the term 'anxiety' going forward. Anxiety is a human condition. It is a complex interplay of our thoughts, emotions, physiology and our behavioural responses. Rest assured, everyone experiences anxiety to some degree. In this book we are confident of educating you on anxiety, and if you or someone you know experiences anxiety to the degree where it is causing suffering and distress, then the PTT approach will provide you with the tools to challenge it and overcome the disabling nature of anxiety.

Anxiety is a general term that covers the full range of anxiety presentations and symptoms, from minor symptoms such as feeling anxious that you will be late for an appointment (and these feelings dissipate once you make it close to the time) or severe anxiety which manifests itself in an actual disorder, such as a phobia, social anxiety or (in Adam's case) OCD. Not all anxiety sufferers will meet the clinical criteria for an anxiety problem, but they may find their symptoms interfere with living and enjoying life. This book is aimed at helping everyone on that spectrum who experiences anxiety.

'Panic' is another term that is often used to describe an anxious state. However, when we use the term, 'panic attack', we are referring to a specific instance in which a person's anxiety symptoms are physically overwhelming but last for a fairly short time. We describe panic attacks in more detail later in the book and in the PTT approach in Part II, but again, panic attacks are another normal human manifestation. They are scary, distressing and become problematic when they occur in what seem like random situations. We may also expect them in situations we fear, such as public speaking, although they are still intensely unpleasant and make us want to avoid any situations which we believe may bring them on. Panic attacks can occur as single events, or as a feature of another anxiety problem. For example, you may suffer from OCD or a phobia, and you will get panic attacks as part of that problem. Or you may just have had a panic attack in response to a single event and it never reoccurs. Or you may have panic attacks as part of Panic Disorder, which is a type of anxiety problem in which the main symptoms are having panic attacks and fearing that they will reoccur. The PTT approach will help you overcome panic attacks whether they happen as standalone events or as part of another problem.

Adam's personal story in Part I of this book sees him overrun and in some cases debilitated by all these issues, but with his primary illness, OCD, leading the charge in his suffering. While I comment a lot on OCD through Adam's story, there is also a lot that is relevant to all anxiety sufferers. Part II of our book is designed for all anxiety sufferers in mind, not just those suffering from OCD. I'm often asked to define OCD and I reply that, at its core, it is **an obsessional problem that can be about absolutely anything, resting on a bed of anxiety, depression, shame and guilt**. There are more commonly occurring types than others, but in summary OCD is when people have intrusive thoughts that are very upsetting, which they interpret to be very threatening, and thus they want to minimise or reduce the threat.[1] Intrusive thoughts are thoughts that are uncontrollable and pop into our heads uninvited. For example, some worrying thoughts may include:

1 Salkovskis, P. M. (1985). Obsessive-compulsive problems: A cognitive-behavioural analysis. *Behaviour Research and Therapy*, 11, 271–7.

- thoughts of deliberately harming yourself or other people
- worries of contamination or catching a disease
- thoughts that you might be a danger to others or yourself in some way
- worries that something bad will happen from something you did or did not do
- fear of disorderliness (i.e. everything must be in its place before you feel content).

The behavioural or compulsive side of these intrusive thoughts is aimed at reducing the perceived threat and feelings of anxiety and might include such things as:

- excessive handwashing and cleaning
- excessive checking and tidying around the house
- repeating words silently
- avoiding people or specific situations
- trying to undo the distressing thoughts in some way
- excessive over-thinking of the worry or possible outcomes

These are just a few of the more common obsessions and compulsions linked with OCD and anxiety, but the first important point to make is that we all have intrusive thoughts. By no means are you alone. We have an estimated 50,000 to 70,000 thoughts a day and we might remember about five of them. And why do we remember those five? Because we've given a meaning to them. That's OCD – when you have a thought that you attach a meaning to, which then allows it to keep intruding in your brain.

For example, you are waiting for a train and suddenly the thought pops into your head, 'What if I jumped in front of the train?' or 'What if I pushed someone in front of the train?' For most people, the thought goes no further than that. But a person with OCD and anxiety might develop the thought along the lines of 'Oh no, I had a thought of killing myself' and then they go on and worry that it means they are suicidal and a danger to themselves. Or they might think, 'Oh no, I'm dangerous to other people' and the meaning or the worry becomes that they want to push someone in front of the train. So they start avoiding trains or buses, or any place they may potentially hurt themselves, or where they could hurt someone else. They avoid visiting friends or relatives, they avoid going to work, they avoid all public places. The intrusive thought is 'I want to harm myself or other people' and the meaning or the worry becomes that they are dangerous; the behavioural or compulsive side is that they must avoid situations in which they could harm themselves or other people. And the more the OCD and anxiety sufferer does to side-step the situation – e.g. avoiding transport, public places etc. – the worse the problem becomes.

The thing about OCD and anxiety is that everything you try and do to reduce anxiety ends up reinforcing the difficulty, thereby creating more anxiety. The more you wash your hands (because you feel unclean and worry you will spread germs), the more you will feel anxious about your potential for infection. The more you worry about stabbing someone, the more you will avoid social situations and subsequently increase your anxiety about them. The more you count the cracks in the pavement (because if you don't, something bad will happen to your family), the more anxious you will become if you fail to do it.

As a therapist, my role is to challenge the meanings of the thoughts that lie behind this illness. By this, I don't necessarily mean analysing them in great depth, trying to figure out where they come from, how they have developed, etc. (although for some people, this can be useful). Instead, I try to get the sufferer to look at each thought in turn, and accept it for what it is – just a thought! This will involve talking through the 'evidence' for the obsession ('I am dangerous, therefore I must avoid all situations in which I could cause harm to myself or others') to get the sufferer to see that what they're obsessing about is only *the thought itself*. It's the thought which is causing the distress, not the so-called 'evidence'.

Once we've challenged the meaning and you've **accepted** that it is a thought, and nothing else, then I'll ask you to look at the unhelpful behavioural and avoidance strategies you are using. Instead of trying to reduce the anxiety by avoiding people, things and situations, we **embrace** the difficulty so that eventually it doesn't bring the crippling anxiety. If you have a fear of germs and you compulsively hand-wash, eventually I might ask you to touch the sole of your shoe with your finger and then put your finger in your mouth. That's going to make 99.9 per cent of all germ-phobics feel very anxious indeed, but each time we do it the anxiety will decrease. With enough exposure, no feeling lasts forever. In this book, Adam will describe how he worried that he might strangle someone. After several sessions I asked him to put his hands around my throat and squeeze. That sounds extreme, but I knew Adam would never actually strangle me. Why? Because it was only *the thought* that was bothering him. When he finally faced his worst fear, he simply withdrew his hands. He **accepted** it was just a thought and we carried on with our session.

There are many types of OCD but at root, the treatment for each type is the same, and it is based on accepting and embracing these thoughts.

Science and psychology haven't pinpointed exactly where OCD and anxiety comes from. There can be an inherited genetic link, but it's by no means guaranteed you will go on and develop OCD. It may be about events as you grow up; perhaps linked to an incident for which you felt responsible, or that you grew up in a house where safety was a constant anxiety. Then again, it can start in your mid-twenties for no apparent reason. As I've mentioned, it isn't entirely necessary that you identify the likely causes as part of your recovery, but for some people (particularly those who ask 'Why me?') it can be useful. You can also get OCD about OCD, and Anxiety about Anxiety, particularly towards the end of treatment. People have had such a distressing time that they worry about the OCD or anxiety coming back. And that's an important part of the recovery process; knowing how to deal with and control those thoughts and worries that threaten to creep in again. I call this the 'maintenance' stage of treatment – maintaining the much-improved mental health you have gained through treatment.

There is also the related **depression**. If OCD and anxiety has taken over your life and you're plagued by worries or thoughts that there is something wrong with you or that you will harm someone, and you're trying desperately to avoid such thoughts and the situations that give rise to such thoughts, then it's no wonder that depression is a factor in this. You start avoiding people and situations; anything you enjoyed doing you won't do any more and you become very self-critical. Well-known models of depression rely on the cutting out of things that give us pleasure, enjoyment or a sense of achievement, and usually an increase in self-criticism. If we have no enjoyment in our life and constantly beat ourselves up, no wonder we feel down!

That said, the trick is to identify which came first, the OCD and anxiety or the depression. If you were clinically depressed before the OCD or anxiety started then you might need treatment for the depression first – possibly a combination of medication and psychological therapy – whereas if depression follows OCD or an anxiety problem then I'd expect it to alleviate as the OCD and anxiety fades. All of this comes down to effective assessment, and I do think this is important before any kind of recovery treatment is embarked upon. If you worry that the depression has been with you longer than the OCD or anxiety, or is so entrenched it might prevent you from being able to take on board this help, then I suggest visiting your doctor to discuss this, and please visit The Shaw Mind Foundation website (www.shawmindfoundation.org) which offers further information and support on all types of mental health problems.

In Part I of this book I will comment on the aspects of Adam's story relating to OCD and anxiety, and describe how we tackled these in his initial therapy sessions with me. In our description of the PTT approach in Part II I will also give you suggestions, exercises and ways of challenging your worries and unpleasant and distressing thoughts so that you can really begin to get a handle on your own condition. It won't always be easy, and there may be times that you will want to seek one-to-one therapeutic advice outside of this book. However, if you do, please make sure that you find someone who understands the **Cognitive Behavioural Therapy and Compassion-Focused Approach** I am outlining. Otherwise, embark upon reading this book and our PTT approach with an open mind and remember that there are millions of people who are struggling just like you. The fact that you've purchased this book means that you have taken the first step towards your recovery. And if you want to, you WILL get better just as Adam did, and he did so at the point when he thought all hope had been lost.

PART I
ADAM'S STORY

My Desperate Struggle with OCD, Anxiety,
Panic Attacks and Related Depression

CHAPTER 1

ADMISSION

Adam: I was in my early thirties and for the third evening in a row I was sitting in the A&E Department at the Northern General Hospital in Sheffield, UK. I'd admitted myself and was desperate for help. If I'd had a physical injury, no doubt I'd have been seen on the first day, treated, and sent home or somewhere else for further treatment. Sadly, it wasn't my body that was playing up; it was my mind. I was going crazy with panic and anxiety attacks, and each time I had a panic attack I didn't think I'd survive the next few minutes.

My sister was with me. My wife, Alissa, and my children were still in Lanzarote (part of the Spanish-owned Canary Islands) where we'd been living for several months. I'd flown home as soon as the signs of anxiety and OCD had crashed into me, but this was worse than anything I'd known in all my years coping with the illness. My sister had found me wandering in the crematorium grounds close to her house and had taken me down to the hospital. She explained to the A&E doctor that I'd had some kind of a mental breakdown and was very poorly. They put me in a room and called out the Mental Health team. Hours later, I was still there, my sister's arms around me as I rocked back and forth in terrible distress.

'What have I done to deserve this?' I thought. 'I've lost control of my life, I'll be admitted to a mental hospital and I won't be able to look after my kids. How have I got to the point where I don't even want to live?'

Still no one came. There were only two members of the Mental Health team on call that night covering the entire city of Sheffield (with a population of more than 550,000) and they were very busy. Eventually, through exhaustion created by hours of intense panic attacks I left and went back to my parents' house, where I was staying while Alissa and the kids were flying home.

And yes, I really felt I didn't want to live. Unbeknown to anyone, and in desperation, the following evening I told my parents I was going out for a walk to try and clear my head.

This was a lie.

In fact, I parked up at a railway bridge close to my home. I climbed onto the bridge and looked down at the track.

'I don't want my kids to see me like this,' I thought.

'Why should their lives be ruined by what's happening to me? I'm of no use to them because I'm in a battle I can't win and one which is consuming me and gradually killing me.'

No trains passed, though several cars drove across the bridge. Nobody stopped. Perhaps they thought I was drunk, or on drugs or something. In hindsight, if someone had stopped or called the police, this may have pushed me to just jump and I might never be writing these words today. It is still very raw and upsetting for me to think about this; that I was in such a desperate place and state of mind that I had lost all hope and this seemed to be the only answer.

What I did not know then was that I was in a severe anxious state of 'Pure O', in which the sufferer has the obsessive thoughts, but not the obvious behavioural compulsions, although I now know that people suffering from Pure O do have mental compulsions, which Lauren later explained to me. Pure O may sound less distressing than OCD, but that couldn't be further from the truth. With Pure O I got to the point where there was nowhere to hide, no safety barrier or technique or compulsion that would help make the state of anxiety subside. It was almost like I was in a 'locked-in' state that I couldn't escape from. The more I tried to get rid of thoughts, the more they would be there and the intensity would increase. By trying to get rid of thoughts, I was making things worse and going against the whole philosophy in this book and the PTT approach of accepting and facing your thoughts and fears.

My whole being was wracked with pain and anxiety, and my emotions were so clouded that I didn't see suicide as a selfish act.

In fact, those contemplating suicide often think the opposite – that those around you and who love you are the selfish ones for implying that suicide is such, because if they knew the pain and distress you are enduring they would let you go and the pain would end, and that they would in fact be better off without you around in your unwell state. Even so, something – perhaps the tiniest glimmer of hope – was telling me that this most destructive of acts was not the way. There had to be something else, a path that would eventually give me peace of mind in this life, not any other, and I believe this tiny bit of hope was driven by thoughts and images of my wife and children. Alissa needed her husband and my children needed their father. I had no say in the matter – I had to get better.

I stepped down from the bridge and got back into the car. I still felt dreadful, pulled apart by panic, anxiety and the most terrible thoughts. Tomorrow I knew I'd be at the hospital again, pleading for the help which I knew the overstretched NHS could not provide there and then. What I didn't know then, but do now, is that there had been such a build-up of OCD and anxiety up to this point in my life that something had to give. It was almost as if my brain had stopped the lifelong fight I'd put up and collapsed in on itself, giving me acute anxiety and panic attacks.

I did go back to the hospital that day, which was almost becoming a compulsion in itself and still there was no help available. But two things happened. The first, while I was sitting there, was a thought which popped into my head – the first rational one I'd had in days.

> *'Adam,'* it said, *'if you ever do recover from this, or find a way through it, you will do something about it and pass it on. You will not recover in silence. You will be public about it, and by exposing it will aim to help other people suffering in the same way. You will make your wife and children proud.'*

The other thing was that I knew I'd have to get myself better. As I've said, I don't blame the NHS for not treating me properly. They're just so under-resourced and overstretched with work that I simply slipped through the net. I was prescribed a medication called diazepam and was told to expect a home visit from the Mental Health team. Then I'd go on to a six-to-twelve-month waiting list for an NHS therapist who might be able to help me. Sadly, I couldn't wait that long; I just knew I needed help much quicker, and that being the case, I'd have to take control and find it myself.

I'd woken up the morning after the bridge incident with ... well, not exactly *motivation*, but something approaching determination to get this sorted once and for all. Alissa and the kids were home and for them, if for no one else, I had to get on my feet and find a way to live without so much anxiety and mental distress.

For the first time – and I'm sure people with OCD and anxiety will not believe me here, but it's true – I logged onto the internet and Googled 'OCD and anxiety'. It had never occurred to me to do it previously; why, I just don't know, but now I think it was an avoidance tactic driven by not wanting to see or hear other sufferers' stories in case my OCD latched onto their obsessions and further increased my internal suffering. Immediately I came across the website for a UK charity called OCD-UK. What I read was nothing short of amazing; I could identify with so many people's stories on so many levels. For years I'd thought I was alone (even though I knew in my heart of hearts that I wasn't). Now I could read the highs and lows of living with OCD and anxiety by real people right across the country. Not that reading about other people's suffering made me feel any better, but at least now I knew that this affects a lot of people around the world and is classed as one of the most debilitating forms of mental illness.

You must understand this: OCD and anxiety is common, and it's not your fault, you have an anxiety or obsessional problem.

I read on, taking in stories of anxiety and related depression. The stories stopped me in my tracks, resonated with me, made me realise we were all in this together. Similar stories, different experiences; they were all there and for the first time I began to realise that my OCD was, if nothing else, at least approachable. So what could I do about it? There was a contact phone number on the website. I rang it and spoke to a man who explained it was a charity.

'I'm in big trouble,' I said. 'I've had this all my life and I'm at a point where I'm suicidal and have lost all hope. I've been to hospital and they don't seem able to help or understand how poorly and desperate I am.'

'Well, Adam,' he replied, 'unfortunately the NHS isn't built to help people with mental illness, especially not the kind which comes on so quickly. So don't feel guilty.'

He told me the only way I'd get immediate access to treatment was to go private. Now, I knew I could afford this. But what if I hadn't been able to? I'd have been in a terrible situation for a long time. So I was, and am, very lucky. For those less able to afford private treatment the situation is dire.

I took down two email addresses. 'They really are the best,' said the man on the phone. I emailed them both, and got responses immediately. They were both based in London. I told them in no uncertain terms that I wasn't fit to travel, and that they'd have to come to Sheffield to see me. One wasn't prepared to do that. Thankfully, the other was, and that's when I first came into contact with Lauren.

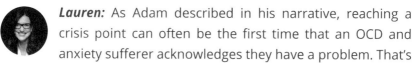 *Lauren:* As Adam described in his narrative, reaching a crisis point can often be the first time that an OCD and anxiety sufferer acknowledges they have a problem. That's not to say they've never been aware of it before – as we will see in the chapters ahead, Adam was fully aware that 'something' was ruining his life, and while he knew what 'it' was, 'it' had attached itself to him so strongly that he was unable to deal with it properly. Instead, he found many ways to avoid 'it' which, in the short term, helped him deal with his unwanted thoughts while he got on with life in the best way he could. In later chapters of Adam's story we will examine these methods of avoidance carefully, but for now let's look at what OCD is and how it might be affecting you.

Let me ask you this: are you having thoughts that are distressing and unwanted? These thoughts could be about fear of catching an illness, or doubts over whether you've locked the door or left the oven on. They might even be about causing harm to yourself and others, or images of bad things happening to people you care for, or carrying out unspeakable acts yourself. Are they causing you distress? If so, what are you doing about them?

If, for example, you have a thought about picking up germs from a door handle and catching a cold (or worse) your next thought might be, 'Oh well, I can catch a cold from anything and anyone. So I might as well just turn the handle and open the door.'

On the other hand, you might think, 'If I touch that door handle and I catch something serious, I could pass it on to my daughter, which could make her really ill or even die. So I must avoid it.'

AND in addition to the last thought, you may also think, 'I may have touched other things around the house that could cause illness. So I'd better wash my hands, and maybe my clothes too, and then clean the house to get rid of any germs.'

The first thought – and millions of others like it – is shared by all of us. Who doesn't have the occasional odd thought about something or someone pop into their head? In OCD these are the **obsessions** that people refer to. Obsessions are persistent and uncontrollable thoughts, images, doubts, fears, impulses and worries. These are also known as **intrusions** because they've suddenly intruded on your everyday thinking. They may also take the form of images, urges or doubts. You might be sitting at your desk and suddenly think of a famous actor or actress. That's normal. You might even search the internet and see what films they have made recently. That's normal too. The thought eventually goes and it becomes just one of the many thousands of thoughts you have every day. This is an example of an intrusive thought as it is uncontrollable and pops into our head uninvited.

But let's say you're at the funeral of your best friend's father and you think of the same famous person. So far, this is normal, though you might be puzzled as to why you're thinking about him or her at such a sad event. Supposing, however, you can't get the image of the famous person out of your head and, worse still, you feel incredibly guilty that you're thinking this way and not focusing fully on the sad occasion. If your friend knew, just imagine how badly he or she would think about you!

This intrusive thought has now become a trigger. You try to push the thought away but it won't go. And the harder you push, the stronger the image becomes.

Now, if this has happened to you before, and you know the only way of getting rid of the thought is, for example, by repeating a prayer, or a certain phrase to yourself, or replacing or undoing the intrusive thought with a 'neutral' or 'safe' thought, then the logical next step is to do that thing. The intrusive thought goes away and you're safe – until the next time it pops into your head and causes you distress. This is Obsessive-Compulsive Disorder (OCD).[2]

As I've said, we all have 'odd' thoughts now and again. They can seem mild or they can seem extreme, but they're just thoughts and they remain that way **until we attach a catastrophic meaning to them**. This last bit is crucial. If we give the thought some importance we're attaching a meaning to it, and so it becomes a trigger. The thought during a funeral about the famous person is of no consequence until you associate it with being a bad friend and start feeling guilty. Similarly, if you encounter someone with a cold and you think, 'I hope I don't catch it,' the thought stays that way until you think, 'I hope I don't catch it because if I do I might pass it to an old person and they could die.' The 'because' bit is the **catastrophic meaning** we attach to it.

This is the 'obsessive' part of OCD. The 'compulsive' or ritualistic part is what you're doing, or not doing, about that thought.

For example, you might be walking over a bridge and you suddenly think, 'Supposing I suddenly jumped over the side of the bridge and into the river?' This is by no means an uncommon thought; we're all human and we're all curious about life, good or bad. But attach a **catastrophic meaning** to that and it becomes, 'I'm thinking about going over the bridge; I must be suicidal and therefore I am dangerous to myself and can't be trusted not to jump off something high.' So you start avoiding bridges, or clifftops and high places in general, and there's your compulsion.

Avoidance is a very big part of OCD, as is seeking reassurance. You have an uncomfortable thought about hurting another person, so you start researching on the internet to see if you have psychopathic tendencies or if you bear the same profile as a serial killer, and you constantly seek reassurance from your partner that they think you

2 Salkovskis, P. M. (1999). Understanding and treating obsessive-compulsive disorder. *Behaviour Research and Therapy*, 37, S29–S52.

are not dangerous. **Avoidance** and **reassurance seeking** in some form are very common compulsions in OCD.

Another part of OCD might be **checking**. You spend around half an hour a day checking that the locks on your front door are working, because you have to be certain that they are locked and multiple checks that they are locked can reassure you to some extent that no one will break in. And every time you walk away from the door, a nagging feeling comes in, which makes you doubt whether you really did lock the door! Even though you are pretty sure you have, it seems safer to you just to check once more …

We all have habits or behaviours that we do to make us feel safe, because it is human nature to have fears, rational or irrational, and then to try and mitigate those fears. What creates OCD are the **catastrophic meanings** you attach to these intrusive thoughts, and what you feel **compelled** to do to ensure something bad doesn't happen. The combinations of these thoughts and behaviours must interfere significantly with your life in some way in OCD. If you have a quick wash of your hands before and after every mealtime and that makes you feel better, then fine. If you're washing your hands for thirty minutes each time until your skin is red raw and other people are noticing, then you have a problem. You can check the door once, but if you're driving home from work several times a day because you're worried you didn't lock it properly, this is going to interfere with living your life.

The example of washing your hands until you feel OK is what we might describe as having a **'just right feeling'** – an arbitrary criterion of deciding when a compulsion can finally stop because it feels 'just right'. For example, if you're washing your hands as described above, only you will know when it feels 'just right' to stop. This could last for any length of time, from a few minutes up to several hours. There is no fixed point because the aim is to get it 'just right'. You're trying to get relief but you're not basing this on anything tangible and it may change constantly. As we will see much later in the book, the way to overcome this is to stop the compulsion when it doesn't feel right, thereby challenging it, which is hard because 'feeling right' is based on a subjective feeling.

In addition, people with OCD and anxiety often feel the need to **confess** unpleasant thoughts they're having and by doing this they get some relief. People will admit to having an uncomfortable thought or carrying out a compulsion (or thought about carrying it out) and their confession becomes a type of compulsion in order to seek reassurance, helping to alleviate anxiety or guilt. We will explore reassurance later in the book and in the PTT approach, and we will see just what an obstacle it is to recovering from anxiety and OCD.

Adam mentions a 'Pure O' form of OCD. This is a term that has become a popular description for people experiencing mental compulsions rather than physical rituals or compulsions or obvious avoidance. They still experience intrusive thoughts, and attach a catastrophic meaning to the thought, but the compulsions are usually done in their head too. This might include 'trying to solve the problem', in your head or repeatedly going over the same worry (**rumination**).

There are many, many variations of OCD; in fact, **you can have OCD about ANYTHING**, but all of them have this in common: an **intrusive thought**, or a trigger; a **catastrophic meaning** that is attached to that thought and **compulsions** or behaviours that help the person temporarily alleviate or avoid the anxiety they feel; and strong, distressing feelings of **anxiety, guilt**, and sometimes **disgust**.

CHAPTER 2

BEGINNINGS

Adam: I was born in the UK in the city of Sheffield in 1977 and raised in Woodseats, a working-class suburb of the city. Our family is a close one; as well as my parents and my sister, I have a large extended family which spends many happy times together.

We were a working-class family – my dad was a builder and my mum worked in a bank. My dad came from one of the poorest parts of Sheffield but he worked hard to build a business and compared to other people in the area we were comfortably off. As a child I enjoyed vacations abroad, nice clothes and brand new sports training shoes. Saying that, my parents made me understand the value of money and how hard work brings rewards in life. So striving for the things I like has never been a shock for me because the work ethic was instilled by my parents.

If I'm asked about my earliest memories I can recall scenes like opening my first-ever Spider-Man toy on Christmas Day, or proudly putting on my new Sheffield Wednesday football kit. Sadly, my strongest memories, which began to form from the age of five, are the ones connected with my developing OCD and anxiety (not that I had any idea I had OCD back then, of course).

My first really debilitating memory stems from my earliest days in school. My mum dropped me off every morning, and just to make sure she wouldn't be knocked down and killed on the way home I began to do little 'rituals'. Quite soon after, I attached these anxious thoughts about my mum to cloud formations. It sounds bizarre, but OCD and anxiety can attach itself to anything. I remember seeing a particular cloud and thinking that if I were the only person to see the cloud my mum would die. So I asked some of my friends to look at the cloud, believing that if they did, it would minimise the risk. Not surprisingly, the anxiety built from there and I dreaded looking into the sky in case I caught a glimpse of a cloud. I begged my mum and dad for a cap that I could wear to school which would prevent me from seeing a cloud, but because I didn't tell them why I wanted it they just thought I was being silly. To this day, there are old schoolmates who remember me saying 'Look at the clouds! Look at the clouds!'

I guess it's funny now, but to a six-year-old it was deadly serious. If I saw those clouds and my classmates didn't, my mum would die, and that felt totally real to me. I felt 100 per cent responsible and accountable for ensuring my mum wouldn't die, something which on reflection is far too much of a burden for a six-year-old. Of course, this took its daily toll on my childhood and therefore my happiness. Perhaps it would have been picked up on now, and something done about it, but back then in the 1980s it was probably seen as slightly odd but otherwise child-like behaviour. Instead, it was the beginning of a journey with OCD and anxiety that would take me to the very darkest of places. This phase went on for a good two or three years before subsiding.

Unfortunately it was replaced by something far more disturbing.

The first time we went to the USA on vacation we were taken to a theme park. As usual, there were queues for all the rides and I remember seeing a disabled boy in a wheelchair who was allowed to go to the front and onto the ride before everyone else.

'Lucky boy,' I thought jealously.

As soon as I had this thought, it came into my head that I was awful for thinking like that. As you would, I suppose, but that thought just wouldn't go away. From then on, every time I saw a disabled person I'd worry excessively that I'd have an evil thought and I worried even more that I'd repeat this out loud to them. At the same time I was anxious about my grandma, who was poorly, and I began to worry that she'd die, and my last thought about her would be a horrible one. So these thoughts about disability, illness, bad thoughts and death became intertwined, and even as we enjoyed the vacation in Florida I was begging my mum not to take me to water parks or even to the Disney parks, so frightened was I that I'd see disabled people and have terrible thoughts about them. At the time, my parents actually just put my actions down to spoilt behaviour for which I was punished.

In short, I was going to great pains to disguise my fears.

This continued back at home. I tried not to see my grandparents and was always on guard for the presence of disabled people. All this avoidance and watching out for triggers was exhausting and depressing too, because I started to avoid things I liked doing for fear of having bad thoughts. I remember seeing footage of the Queen Mother on TV and being terrified that I'd think a bad thought about her and she'd die the day after. From then on, I couldn't face seeing or hearing anything about the Queen Mother.

And yet I was a popular child, with plenty of friends. I wasn't a loner or particularly unusual, outwardly at least. Neither did I have a difficult childhood. In fact, if the OCD and anxiety had disappeared I'd have been the happiest, most well-balanced kid around. And this continued into secondary school. I was good at sport, particularly basketball and football, and I was captain of these teams. Yet under the surface I was a complete mess and for no apparent reason other than extreme anxiety. The perceived constant battle in my head was energy-sapping and soul-destroying.

My OCD and anxiety distracted me so much at secondary school that I left with just two GCSE qualifications. I was seen as not being particularly academic, but in fact, I was clever enough. I just didn't put in the work because I was spending so much time staring out of the window, trying to manage the obsessive thoughts running through my brain on a loop for most parts of the school day. I didn't want people to know I was a worrier, so it seemed easier to simply disengage and pretend I was struggling academically, both to friends and family. What I didn't know then was that by avoiding it, running away and disengaging, I was simply fuelling it.

The obsessions became worse. I went from thinking I'd swear at disabled people to being terrified that I'd actually hurt vulnerable people, particularly the elderly and young children. I remember hearing and reading about the James Bulger killing (in which two ten-year-old boys from Liverpool were convicted of the 1993 murder of a three-year-old boy). There was public outrage throughout the UK and almost overnight I talked myself into believing that I too would become a child killer. There were a couple of young boys living round the corner from me and I was sure that one day I'd strangle them. It got to the point that I didn't dare to be around young children in case I led them off and killed them. Items on the news about shootings, stabbings, severe mental illness or people with schizophrenia murdering people used to disturb me deeply, keeping me awake most nights as I'd believe I would do the same to someone else. I was absolutely torturing myself with such thoughts, but couldn't tell anyone. My parents noticed that I wasn't doing as much sport but they put it down to me becoming a bit lazy as I went into teenagehood. It was becoming a huge battle to find the motivation to put on a mask to my parents, and anyone else who might have noticed I was behaving oddly. In fact, it was exhausting.

Funnily enough, the kids at school didn't notice, perhaps because on occasions I was putting my obsessions and compulsions to good use. For example, I would practise basketball shots again and again and again until I got them right. And so I stood out in a positive way. Unfortunately, my schoolwork and academic aspirations went in the other direction, as I've described. Perhaps the will to succeed in some areas was driven by the fear of failure, and I've always had a natural drive to be the best. My OCD pushed me on to succeed (and I do try to look for positives!) but as I grew up and left school the illness threatened to overwhelm me completely, extracting a very heavy price.

 Lauren: A question I'm often asked by clients is: '*How and why did my OCD or anxiety problem start?*' It's an interesting question, and although we don't need the answer to learn how to manage OCD or an anxiety problem, we're all human and we like to solve mysteries. It's also important to stress that not all adults with OCD had OCD as children. It can develop in adulthood too so you don't need to have had childhood OCD or anxiety in order for it to come on in later life. Similarly, not all anxious adults experienced anxiety as children. Likewise with an anxiety disorder, not all anxious adults had an anxiety problem starting in childhood. However, there is evidence that an untreated anxiety problem or OCD in childhood will then continue in to adulthood. In summary, we cannot pick exactly who will develop an anxiety problem or OCD.

Research suggests that both anxiety problems and OCD have biological and psychological origins and can combine with external factors to trigger illness. OCD and anxiety can run genetically in families, with varying degrees of susceptibility to it. However, in some cases it is very clear why an anxiety problem or OCD has developed. For example, in the case of a phobia of dogs, the person had a traumatic experience a few years before which involved being chased by a Rottweiler dog. Or in the case of OCD, a new mother has intrusive thoughts about harming her baby and then went on to develop OCD. When I'm assessing a patient before treatment I will take a holistic view of them, their background and how they view their experiences in life. The latter can give the most significant clues; as I said in Chapter I, **it is not the worry that counts, but the catastrophic meanings we have attached to that thought or experience**.

You may already have a good idea about how and why your OCD or anxiety problem developed, or you may be reading this book thinking, 'Why me? I don't have a clue why OCD or anxiety picked on me!' If you think about the time that your OCD or anxiety problem developed, you may find some clues – did something significant happen at the time? Were you feeling more stressed than usual? Or are there certain rules or ways of living that you grew up with that you think may have contributed to your OCD or anxiety problem? However, even if you are still unsure of why your OCD or anxiety problem developed, rest assured we don't need to uncover this in order for you to get better.

In cases of Childhood OCD, which Adam suffered from, the OCD trigger might be something very simple. For example, a child has mislaid his school jumper after PE. The child's mum has emphasised how important it is to look after his things, perhaps with the implication that something bad will happen if he doesn't. So the child places meaning on that implication and it becomes a reality – *'If I don't do something (in this case, look after my things), something terrible will happen.'* As a child, you might accidentally touch some dog faeces. That's a horrible thing to happen to anyone, but if a child attaches meaning to it (*'That's dirty, and I'm dirty for touching it'*) that can lead to contamination OCD. The difficulty we can have is that sometimes it is hard for a child to actually tell us what they are worried about, or even make sense of it themselves. This is very normal, and we cover this issue in great detail in our Juniors and Teenagers Edition of Pulling the Trigger (www.pulling-the-trigger.com).

In Adam's case, he was worrying about his mum dying. He looked up and saw a cloud, then attached a meaning to the thought about his mum dying, i.e. that if he was the only one to see that cloud, his mum would die. So what is a normal worry for a child suddenly becomes an obsession, and a compulsion develops from it. It's also normal for children to develop habits, but when these habits become something which causes distress we can be pretty sure we might have a problem with OCD or anxiety. As a parent, you might see a behavioural disturbance, avoidance, or physiological signs manifest themselves first. As we mentioned, children (especially young children) can't always articulate their worries so instead you might see behaviours, including:

- avoidance of things they used to do
- seeking reassurance
- sleep problems
- physical complaints, including headaches and stomach aches
- increased irritability and tearfulness
- becoming more clingy
- school refusal

With childhood OCD you may see more ritualised behaviour including;

- switching lights on and off
- checking locks and taps
- repetitive handwashing or excessive showering

- counting rituals, often at bedtime
- refusing to let go of old or apparently useless items
- requests for family members to repeat phrases or answer the same question.

These are only a selection of behaviours and changes. You might think that many of them go hand-in-hand with 'normal' childhood behaviour. And you'd be right, except that it's possible the anxious child believes:

- *that something bad is going to happen*

And in particular with OCD they may believe:

- *doing this makes me feel better, and less anxious*.

As parents, what can we do about anxiety and OCD in children? With anxious children, it is important to follow a guided approach in helping children overcome their anxiety problem. If they do not receive help, then it is likely that not only will they continue to believe their worries, but they can develop long term anxiety problems that continue into adulthood.

With children you suspect are suffering from OCD, my advice would be to intervene. Interfere with the ritual and see what happens. For example, don't let your child switch the lights on and off a number of times. If it causes distress, ask your child what she/he is worrying about and see if you are able to put their fears into context. It is important to tackle it. Don't accommodate it, because a child can attach extra meaning to the fact you recognise the behaviour and are allowing it to continue. Even if you make your child feel uncomfortable, albeit temporarily, it's important that you intervene to stop the behaviour before it becomes worse.

Sometimes children with OCD don't know why they engage in the rituals or compulsions, only that it makes the anxiety go away. You can still challenge the compulsion by setting up experiments to test what will happen – will the uncomfortable feeling go away if you don't do the compulsion? Once a child realises that the anxiety feeling eventually goes away, they are usually open to challenging more of the OCD and anxiety and doing more experiments. As I mentioned, we discuss childhood OCD and anxiety in our Juniors and Teenagers

Edition of Pulling the Trigger so please refer to this for further help and support on childhood anxiety (www.pulling-the-trigger.com).

If you're an adult with OCD or an anxiety problem reading the above, you might recognise some or all of these behaviours and as I said at the beginning, it may be very helpful to discover an 'explanation' for your OCD or anxiety problem. You may have also seen how these behaviours have acted as a 'friend', both in Adam's life and yours. The little behaviours you performed as a child were a kind of 'comfort blanket'. They helped you feel in control and reduced your anxiety. However, none of us can change or 'fix' the past. If you're still holding on to such beliefs, or you can see how they've grown and taken new shape over the years, now is the time to look at them in more depth and consider what these beliefs mean for you today.

CHAPTER 3

AIR CRASH

Adam: After school and at the age of sixteen I went to the local college to study for a qualification in Sports Management. Sport was what I liked doing best, so it seemed sensible to follow that career path. Also, it got me outside in a competitive environment, and away from my thoughts.

Happily, my mind calmed down a little during those years. There was plenty to distract me – sport, new friends, alcohol, nights out – and so the first few months at college were comfortable. That said, anxiety and a constant morbid awareness of my mindset always lurked in the background and never seemed far from reappearing. I remember once holding a pen and feeling that I would stab the boy sat next to me with it. So I stopped holding a pen in class and got in trouble for not doing any work. When my parents heard about it they thought I was being lazy. The truth was that I just couldn't pick up a pen for fear of harming people, and somehow I managed to persuade my friends to help me out with written work.

I should say now that I'm not, and never have been, a violent person. Being tall and good at sport I could stick up for myself and I occasionally ended up in minor scuffles and fights at school, but I never provoked anyone and certainly never went out looking for trouble. I was a normal kid who didn't like being pushed around, but was respectful of other people and wasn't a troublemaker. Perhaps that's why I was so anxious about having violent thoughts – the very idea of hurting someone deliberately was appalling to me, so it preyed on my mind.

I met a girl at college who became my girlfriend and almost overnight the OCD and anxiety went away. She was my first proper girlfriend and when you're young you put all your emotions into new relationships.

Now I see that our relationship was my biggest distraction to date, which served as avoidance for my OCD and anxiety. At the time I just thought I'd got better. I had no nasty intentions towards her and even though I worried that the anxiety and obsessions would return, if I ever did have an unpleasant thought it would be like anyone else's unpleasant thought – over and done with in a second.

So life seemed OK. There was only one incidence of OCD when I was with my girlfriend, and that was when we were on vacation in Cyprus. We went out for a meal one night and I was eating meatballs with a fork. For a moment, the thought entered my head that I might stab her with the fork. I put down the utensil, and from then until the rest of the vacation I made excuses not to go to restaurants, instead making sure we ate at fast-food places where you could use your fingers. It sounds silly, but I was frightened of what I might do and wanted to avoid any situations that would trigger the thoughts.

From a young age, probably since my family started going abroad on vacation, I'd been very interested in aircraft and flying. Although I hadn't done well at school and was on a Sports Management course, my real dream was to be a qualified pilot. When I was feeling poorly in school I promised myself that if I ever got better I'd learn to fly. Although I eventually broke up with my girlfriend, my fears and anxieties had been relatively calm for some time and I thought I was in a place where I was making progress. I sat down with my parents and told them about my dream.

'OK, Adam,' my dad said, 'if you want to get your pilot's licence you'll have to work to pay for it. If you get a job and save up half the cost, we'll pay the other half.'

It was a deal. I got a job in a local pizza restaurant and worked all hours so that I could pay for the course. I applied myself to getting my licence like I'd never applied myself to anything before. I was utterly determined. I flew a Cessna 152 light aircraft from Netherthorpe Airfield in South Yorkshire, and as I was building up my flying hours I was also working towards the theory exams. When I finally took the papers, I passed all twelve Private Pilot's Licence (PPL) exams first time. My parents were surprised, to say the least.

'It seems like you just didn't try hard enough at school, did you Adam?' said my mum.

'It's probably true,' I replied. 'I was a bit immature back then.' But I couldn't tell her the real reason – that I was too busy trying to control my thoughts to concentrate on studying.

Now all that had disappeared, I didn't need to tell her anything.

I felt so good by now that once I'd passed my PPL I wanted to train to become an airline pilot. The course would cost £60,000, it was based in Oxford and no one in my family had ever considered doing anything like this before. It was a big step but I was more than prepared to take it. I took out a loan for the money, which my mum and dad secured for me, got onto the course and moved to Oxford. I needed to pass more exams – eighteen papers in total – to get through the first stage of the course, including maths and physics. I was determined and passed them easily. These exams are incredibly tough and very demanding academically. To go from two GCSE qualifications to passing the Airline Transport Pilot's Licence (ATPL) exams first time with a high percentage pass rate demonstrates how I'd allowed OCD and anxiety to affect my life at school. It was easier to let everyone assume I was academically challenged. Just three people out of the twenty-four-strong cohort passed first time, including me, and many of these candidates had been picked from university by British Airways.

The next part of the course was learning how to fly commercial airliners, which took place in Arizona. I needed to put in 250 hours' flying time to get a 'frozen' ATPL, which meant I'd be able to work for an airline. Then I would be able to take my flying time up to 1,500 hours to get an active ATPL. Arizona was wonderful. I loved the flying, the surroundings, the friends I was making on the course.

It was all going well. Too well, in fact ...

In a life dominated by OCD and anxiety I've noticed that when things are really going my way and I feel there is nothing getting in my way of reaching my goals, suddenly something kicks in and my mental health issues begin to really knock me back. And so it did in Arizona. One day I was heading for the airfield with the intention of flying a turbo-prop aircraft. I passed through reception, and as I did so I noticed the young receptionist at the desk, a girl I'd seen occasionally before.

'I'm going to strangle her,' I thought.

It came right out of the blue, and no sooner had it done so than it lodged in my brain, gripped tight and wouldn't let go. The thought horrified me and my anxiety went sky high.

'I'm going to strangle her. It must mean I'm likely to do this, therefore I'm dangerous, they will arrest me and put me in a mental hospital or prison here in Arizona. I will never see my family or friends again in the UK.'

'I'm going to strangle her. I'm £60,000 in debt and my career is over. My parents are the guarantors of my loan, they will lose the family home and everything they have ever worked for because their son is an evil murderer.'

'I'm going to strangle her. I can't get that thought out of my head and it will drive me mad.'

'I'm going to strangle her. It's such an awful thought that it must mean that I really want to do this; there is no getting away from this.'

I didn't fly that day, or any day after that. I just turned around, went back to my room, and lay in bed for two days. I begged my brain to remove the thought, but it wouldn't go. My classmates rallied round and wondered what was wrong. I told them my dad was ill and I was feeling a bit down. In my heart, I knew I'd messed up big time. This thought was not going away, and there was no chance of me getting into a cockpit. I was a danger to myself and others. At least that's what I thought.

I was terribly anxious about ringing my parents. They had to know I wasn't well, and that I needed to come home. All sorts of thoughts swirled around my brain: 'How can I explain to them that I might be a psychopath?' 'Will they disown me because something is mentally wrong with me?' 'How will I repay the money they've lent me?' 'What will I do next?'

The thought of speaking to them filled me with fear and horror, but I had to do it. I rang home and mum answered.

'Hi Adam!' she said brightly, 'How are you doing?'

'Mum, I'm not very well …' I began.

Her tone changed immediately. 'Why?' she said, sounding serious.

'What's wrong?'

I tried to pretend, tried to say I was getting bad headaches and couldn't concentrate. She replied that they'd be gone in a day or so, and not to worry. I tried again, this time telling her that 'something wasn't right with my head'.

I'm not sure she really understood that, but she became very quiet. I could hear my dad in the background asking, 'What's wrong? What's wrong? Does he need to come home?'

'I think you do need to come home, don't you Adam?' she said. 'Don't worry, we'll sort it out.'

I just sobbed and sobbed. Telling them was the hardest thing I'd ever had to do. Instinctively they knew something was seriously wrong, and they booked a flight for me the following day.

My friends took me to the airport. They hugged me and put comforting arms round my shoulders.

'See you when your dad's better!' they said.

I smiled and returned the hugs, knowing I'd never see them again and that my life was over.

Some of them kept in touch, but even now they think my dad had a heart attack and I couldn't continue the course for that reason.

I don't know how I managed to get on that plane. I was wracked with anxiety and guilt, and my brain and body felt totally separate. Somehow I managed it, curling up into my seat in the hope that no one would think that I looked strange. The thoughts of strangling people kept coming and coming, a powerful feeling that forced me to sit on my hands for the entire eleven-hour flight.

'Don't have an urge,' I whispered to myself. 'Don't have an urge, don't have an urge, don't have an urge …' As we touched down back in the UK, I released my hands from underneath me, they were completely numb and felt lifeless. I struggled to even grab my bag from the overhead baggage compartment as the sensations of pins and needles began to kick in. As I exited the aircraft I felt drained of all my energy and appetite simply from trying to prevent any urges during the long flight.

Mum picked me up at the airport. I was white as a sheet. I hardly spoke on the journey home up the motorway. All I could think about was how 'this' had finally got me, ruined my career, left me £60,000 in debt. Back then, you could buy a nice house in Sheffield for that kind of money. It was the first time I seriously considered throwing myself under a train so I could relieve myself of the anguish and the perceived mess I had created. I felt I wasn't fit to be around other people, never mind fly a planeload of them around the world. In the past I'd kept my thoughts at bay with distractions, but this time it had completely bypassed everything. My life was over.

 Lauren: A friend told me about a balloon flight she'd had. It was her third flight, so she'd had a reasonable amount of experience in take-off, landing and how it felt when the balloon was in flight, hundreds of feet up.

'It was a beautiful evening,' she said, 'with just enough wind to push us along. As we floated across the hills all of the land and sky seemed at peace. Then this thought entered my head: *"What if I were to just sit on the edge of the basket and push myself off?"* It was just one of those silly thoughts, but it stayed with me and I wondered what might've happened had I taken it seriously ...'

A 'silly thought', just one of the estimated 50,000 to 70,000 thoughts we have every day. Not all of them are silly: some are for problem-solving, others are practical. Some might be nostalgic, repetitive, intelligent, stupid, creative, dull – the variations are huge. And yes, some of them might seem totally bizarre to us, like the one about pushing yourself over the side of the basket of a balloon.

The latter thought was what we would describe as an **intrusive** one. At 1,000 feet up, it was a thought that wasn't particularly welcome at that point, fanciful though it was. It was a thought that might make you question why it popped into your head. Luckily for my friend, she mused about it and then let it go. She has said she will go ballooning again – so problem over.

But what if that thought HAD stayed with her? What if she'd gone home that night and been unable to push the thought away? And, worse still, what if that thought had led her to question her motives, and even her sanity? What if she'd come to believe that she'd had a suicidal thought and therefore there was something seriously wrong with her? She might never have flown in a balloon again, and she might have avoided bridges over rivers and railways, or any other high places, for fear she would jump. Her life would have become difficult as a result. That is what can happen when we attach a **catastrophic meaning** to an intrusive thought. This is what happens when people develop OCD.

For example, let's look at this thought. *'Tomorrow, my partner/child/ mother/father is going to die in a crash.'* That's an upsetting thought, but it is a normal one. However, it is one that is very hard to repeat to oneself – even among psychologists and therapists – because the meaning we infer when we say it to ourselves is that **somehow it might happen BECAUSE we have said it might**. The fact that it's 99.9999 per cent unlikely to happen has little or no relevance; we've already attached a meaning to it, and that is what counts to us.

The 'meaning' side of OCD has three parts; the first is the **catastrophic interpretation** ('What's the worst that could happen?'), then the **blame** side comes ('I've had this terrible thought and it's my fault if something happens'). The last part is the **duty** we put upon ourselves to try and stop the bad thing or prevent it from happening ('I've had this thought, but there is something I can do to control it, or make it go away').[3]

Let's look at Adam's intrusions and meanings in his account. Firstly, he's having a meal with his then girlfriend. He picks up a fork and thinks, 'I could stab her with this ...' This is the **intrusive thought**.

3   Salkovskis, P. M., Wroe, A. L., Gledhill, A., Morrison, N., Forrester, E., Richards, C., Reynolds, M., Thorpe, S. (2000). Responsibility attitudes and interpretations are characteristic of obsessive compulsive disorder. *Behaviour Research and Therapy*, 38(4), 347–72.

OK, it's not a pleasant thought, but here's a secret … not everyone's thoughts are 100 per cent lovely all the time! In fact, we all have dark thoughts occasionally. We wouldn't be human if we didn't. Everyone has occasional thoughts along the lines of, 'I could murder that traffic warden/cold caller/doorstep salesman' etc. But most of us attach no significance to it. We let the thought go – end of story.

But when Adam picked up that fork and had an intrusive thought about how he would use it, he allowed that thought to dominate.

In other words, he gave it **a catastrophic meaning** and it became troublesome. The fear of the thought forced him to avoid restaurants, and other places he might come across a similar utensil, just in case he had the thought again. As we will see later on, the very act of avoidance gave power and even greater meaning to the thought.

As part of the **catastrophic meaning** that Adam attached to the thought, he also interpreted the thought as meaning that either deep down in his subconscious he really wanted to stab her, as evidenced by having such an awful thought, or that he was at risk of doing such an awful thing. This type of thinking is known as **Thought-Action Fusion**; that having such a thought means it is more likely to happen, or that it means that thinking about the action is as bad as actually doing it.[4]

Another devastating thought Adam experiences in this chapter happened during his flying training. He sees the receptionist at the aerodrome and thinks: 'I'm going to strangle her.'

An intrusive thought, yes. But nonetheless, just a thought … until he attaches meaning to it. This is how he describes his thought process:

(*Intrusive Thought*) **'I'm going to strangle her.'**

(*Catastrophic Meaning*) **'I can't get that thought out of my head and it will drive me mad.'**

(*Intrusive Thought*) **'I'm going to strangle her.'**

(*Catastrophic Meaning*) **'I'm £60,000 in debt and my career is over. My parents are the guarantors of my loan, they will lose the family home and everything they have ever worked for because their son is mentally unwell.'**

4   Rachman, S. (1997). A cognitive theory of obsessions. *Behaviour Research and Therapy*, 35, 793–802.

(*Intrusive Thought*) **'I'm going to strangle her.'**

(*Catastrophic Meaning*) **'It must mean I'm likely to do this, therefore I'm dangerous; people will eventually find out, arrest me and put me in a mental hospital or prison.'**

(*Intrusive Thought*) **'I'm going to strangle her.'**

(*Catastrophic Meaning*) **'It's such an awful thought that it must mean that I really want to do this.'**

Do you see what's going on here? Adam attaches a variety of **catastrophic meanings** to his initial thought, and each one becomes increasingly calamitous. He cannot control his intrusive thought, in exactly the same way that none of us can. However, he has chosen to respond to it in a way that is going to cause him a problem. As it turns out, the **catastrophic meanings** he attaches to that thought will actually change his life.

We all have intrusive thoughts. It's how we choose to interpret them which determines whether they will become a problem for us.

Adam's desperate attempts to control his thoughts, to push them aside, invent rituals to suppress them or avoid situations in which they may occur, actually make his problems worse. He takes his intrusive thought very seriously, and in doing so gives it a **catastrophic meaning** – and therefore makes it powerful.

People can have intrusions about all sorts of things: becoming unwell, carrying out strange sexual acts, contaminating themselves and other people, causing harm to others, being responsible for fires or floods, cheating on their partner, causing God to become angry – anything at all that can be considered an intrusive thought. All these thoughts are normal – it's the **catastrophic meaning** we attach that gives them importance.

But we don't just have intrusive thoughts in OCD. We can have intrusions in any anxiety or obsessional problem. What makes it more confusing is that we can also have intrusive images, urges, doubts, or sensations. For example, you are out jogging and you suddenly notice a pain down your arm – this is an intrusive physical sensation. You are about to give a presentation at work and just beforehand you have an intrusive image pop into your head of yourself making a mistake or blushing during the presentation. You are standing on the train station platform and you have an intrusive urge to throw yourself in front of the next train. You are at the airport about to fly off on a well-deserved vacation and you have intrusive doubts whether you actually sent those emails to clients before leaving the office. All these are types of intrusions, uncontrollable and seemingly come from out of the blue.

We can have intrusive thoughts, images, sensations, doubts or urges about anything. Some of these may occur in the presence of an anxiety or obsessional problem, or some may just occur as one-off events. If you notice the physical sensation in your arm while out jogging, you may attach a **catastrophic meaning** to it; 'I am having a heart attack or likely to have one', and therefore may take yourself to the hospital and stop jogging all together, or doing any other form of exercise. If you have images of yourself blushing or making a mistake in your presentation to your colleagues, you may have attached a **catastrophic meaning**; 'I am going to look stupid, everyone will notice that I am blushing and I will be embarrassed', and you may have a number of behaviours that you do in order to stop this feared outcome such as wearing makeup, making sure you are wearing loose clothing so you don't get too hot and red in the face and making the presentation as short as possible. When you are standing on the train platform waiting for the train, you give a **catastrophic meaning** to the urge that 'I must want to kill myself' and thus start avoiding train platforms and no longer take the train. At the airport you give a **catastrophic meaning** to the doubts that you had sent important emails; 'I didn't get those emails off to clients, so I will be in trouble with my boss and lose out on the commission', and therefore you ring your colleagues in the office to check on your behalf that the emails have been sent.

These examples could be part of an anxiety or obsessional problem, including:

- Panic Disorder;
- Social Anxiety Disorder;
- Health Anxiety Disorder;

- Generalised Anxiety Disorder;
- Obsessive Compulsive Disorder.

However, if you have an intrusion, and you attach a **catastrophic meaning** and it doesn't change your behaviour considerably, then it may be a stand-alone event that although it caused you anxiety on that specific day, does not indicate an anxiety problem. For example, in the jogging situation, if you notice the sensations in your arm, and you have the thought 'I could be having a heart attack', and might decide to check it out with your GP later that week and you continue jogging the next day. Even though it caused anxiety on the first day it did not escalate into a problem. Equally, if you are at the airport and have doubts about work emails, attach the **catastrophic meaning** and even if you ask your colleagues to check for you, this incident has only happened once in five years so it is not likely to be an anxiety problem. The severity of the interference in our life of these events is key in diagnosing an anxiety problem. If it interferes for one day, then never again, it is unlikely to have become an anxiety problem. If, however, it starts to interfere on one day and we continue to change our behaviours, including avoiding things such as taking the train or doing any exercise, then it is likely to have become an anxiety problem.

When I talk to clients about anxiety and the responses they do in order to prevent the feared outcome from happening I use a scale to show where thoughts and behaviours would be considered 'clinically diagnosable' as an anxiety problem. The anxiety problem has to 'significantly interfere' in your life to be considered diagnosable. For example, in the jogging situation, if you notice the pain in your arm and stop jogging for only one day due to the worry of having a heart attack, then you would not be diagnosed with an anxiety problem and would be lower down the scale. However, if the incident caused you to worry about having a heart attack on a daily basis and you now avoid not only jogging but all forms of exercise, then you are likely to have a diagnosable anxiety problem.

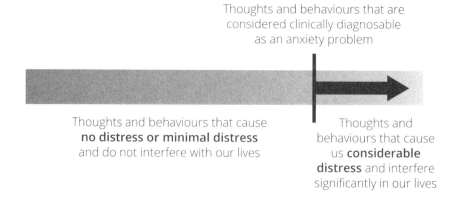

Figure 1: Scale showing differing severity of anxiety interfering thoughts and behaviours.

Likewise when I talk to clients about OCD obsessions and compulsions I would use the same scale, to show where thoughts and behaviours become ones we might categorise as OCD. Here is the scale:

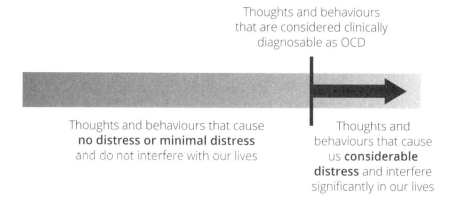

Figure 2: Scale showing differing severity of OCD thoughts and behaviours.

So, at the bottom end of the scale are thoughts and behaviours that do not cause distress or interfere much in our life. As we go up the scale we see the thoughts and behaviours are causing us more distress and interfering much more in our daily living. As professionals, we have to have some classification for knowing when someone is 'diagnosed' with OCD or an anxiety problem. Each anxiety problem or obsessional problem has it's own criteria. For example, in the case of OCD we have decided that is when these obsessions and compulsions are causing that person significant distress and take up more than one hour a day. Hence, the mark in the graph indicates that when you have moved over into this area you would be considered 'diagnosable' with OCD. Even if you are still on the other side, the non-diagnosable side, it still might be that your obsessions and compulsions are causing you distress, albeit less frequently or less severely than those diagnosed with OCD. However, it doesn't matter. Treatment can help people at any point on this scale.

In addition, you will not stay at a fixed place on the scale – you can move up and down it depending on your symptom severity and how much it is interfering in your life. For example, when Adam had a severe episode of anxiety he was almost at the top of the scale. As he felt better, during and following therapy, he moved down the scale. You may have a 'blip' during or after treatment that forces you back up the scale for a short time, but then by using the strategies in this book and our recovery approach contained within it, you can quickly bring yourself back down the scale. You may always be on the scale at some place, but this place can vary and you can keep yourself on the 'non-diagnosable' side.

Still unsure of whether you have an anxiety problem? Let me ask you some questions:

- Do you worry a lot about a particular situation or event?
- Do you worry more than other people?
- Do you worry about lots of things most of the time?
- Do your worries stop you doing things or going places?
- Do you make efforts to avoid particular situations or events because of how anxious you feel or out of worry of what might happen if you didn't avoid them?
- Do you have specific things you have to do to stop the feared outcome from happening?
- Do you find it difficult to control your worry?
- Do you feel nervous, anxious, on edge?

- Do you feel physically stressed? (for example, you may have a sore back, headaches, upset stomach or digestive problems)
- Do you worry something bad might happen?
- Do you have trouble sleeping?
- Do you have trouble relaxing?

Specifically related to OCD, let me ask you some more questions:

- Do you have unpleasant thoughts, images or doubts that repeatedly enter your mind?
- Do you worry excessively about terrible things happening?
- Do you have concerns about acting on an unwanted and senseless urge or impulse?
- Do you feel driven to perform certain acts over and over again? (This may include checking, confessing, counting, examining your body for signs of illness or anxiety, touching things, repeating actions, collecting objects, arranging things, washing and cleaning.)
- Do you avoid people, places or things in case they trigger unwanted thoughts or urges?
- Do you seek comfort or reassurance from others (family or professionals) or from the internet that there is nothing wrong with you or that bad things are unlikely to happen?

If you said 'yes' to some of these questions, it might mean you have OCD or another anxiety disorder. However, some, all or none of this may apply to you, but please keep reading. It might be the case that you are still at the point where your behaviour is keeping you 'safe' for the moment and that you are not experiencing many obsessions or worries, or having to do many compulsions or other 'safe' behaviours. However, such 'safe' behaviour has a tendency to escalate, in that you need to carry out more and more 'safe' behaviours to make yourself feel better. Or it has become so normal to do these 'safe' behaviours that you don't even consider them as part of the problem. In the next chapter we will look at these 'safe' behaviours, compulsions and rituals and how they are detrimental in the long term.

CHAPTER 4

THE KEYS TO MY ANXIETY

Adam: So I was home, but still very poorly. Far from the anxieties and fears of hurting people disappearing, they seemed stronger than ever. Again, I tried to explain the inner workings of my head to my parents, leaving out the 'killing' part, but it was probably all coming out wrong. My dad wanted me to go to the St Wilfrid's Centre in Sheffield to seek some kind of advice and support; it was a church-based organisation that helped vulnerable people, particularly the homeless and those with mental health issues. I had – and have – nothing against such people but I didn't fit into the 'homeless' category.

The fear of being sent to St Wilfrid's added fuel to my anxiety. What if I ended up there, and harmed a disabled or homeless person? I would be a murderer, and the worst kind of murderer because I'd killed someone vulnerable. I'd be locked up forever and I'd deserve everything I'd get. The thoughts went round and round, tormenting me day and night. My parents must have been in complete despair as I was just not responsive to any communication. I was on autopilot, consumed and drained by highly anxious thoughts and out of touch with what was going on around me.

Finally, I was persuaded to see my local doctor. My mum took me and sat outside in the waiting room while I went in. I tried to explain to the doctor how I felt and what was going on in my head. He listened, umm'd and ahhh'd, then delivered his expert opinion:

'Perhaps you should just stop worrying and go for a nice walk in the park,' he said. 'That might clear it all up.'

I could have cried. He just didn't understand at all. Mind you, a bit of fresh air was nice, I have to admit, and besides, I'd already found a way to get rid of the murderous thoughts. I figured that I could somehow bind my hands if I had a thought of strangling someone in a public place, so I went to a local military surplus shop and invested in a pair of handcuffs. I kept these in my pocket, deciding that if I ever had an overwhelming need to kill (particularly someone vulnerable, like a woman or a child) I could ask the nearest person to simply put the handcuffs on me.

Now, imagine that scenario in practice. It sounds ridiculous, the kind of bizarre incident you'd read about in the papers. But to me, it was a very serious situation and only an extreme way of dealing with it could put my mind at rest.

I had the handcuffs in my pocket one afternoon as I took a walk close to my home, about two weeks after I returned from Arizona. Across the road was a girl I recognised, the daughter of some friends of my parents. I waved to her and crossed the road to speak to her. It was a while since I'd seen her. We chatted, and it transpired she wanted to move out of her home and find an apartment. As it happened, my parents had a place to rent and so Alissa moved in, to everyone's satisfaction. She was a lovely and very attractive girl, and both sets of parents were close. In the weeks that followed I kept bumping into her and after a while we starting seeing each other as boyfriend and girlfriend.

'Now,' you might ask, 'what business did he have with a girlfriend when he was having so many bad thoughts about killing people?' It's a fair question, and I can only answer it this way: the thoughts I had felt real to me and I had now found a way of dealing with them. Besides, I didn't have the slightest intention of harming Alissa. On the contrary, I was falling in love with her and after being in such a bad place was relieved that finally I seemed to be finding happiness, as I had never been in love before.

Maybe I should have asked myself then why I had no intention of harming Alissa and yet had felt that way in general? Perhaps I didn't want to break the spell; the one that I'd just fallen under which seemed to be taking away my fears and bringing back my contentment. Alissa was younger than me, but we knew we were right for each other. Nothing else seemed to matter, least of all my anxieties. And soon Alissa became pregnant; she was my life and I was really happy.

It was time to accept my responsibilities, prepare for fatherhood and put my troubled past behind me.

That said, there were fears around the birth of the baby which still troubled me. I wondered if the thoughts of harming would attach themselves to my child. It was a niggling worry, and a scary one. I knew I didn't feel that way about Alissa. But might I feel differently towards the baby? As ever, I distracted myself by pushing the thoughts right to the back of my mind. I really couldn't go there.

I couldn't go back to flying. I was still heavily in debt to my parents and there was no way I'd return to Arizona now – and incur any more debt. So I applied for and got a job at an insurance company called Aon which was working on behalf of the British government dealing with compensation claims by former British coal miners suffering from chronic pulmonary diseases. I was happy in my work, and even happier with my domestic arrangements. I had a job, a baby on the way and I was in love. I was becoming a 'normal' person at last.

Our daughter was born and, as with the birth of anyone's first child, life changed considerably. We adjusted to being parents in the best way we could and I was working hard at Aon to provide for my family. Going home wasn't much of a relief, as anyone with a new baby knows. Stress and general fatigue can make OCD and anxiety thrive and during this time I found my levels were higher than normal. Luckily, my anxiety hadn't attached to our firstborn, in that I had no thoughts about harming her. Unfortunately, the thoughts around harming had entered a new phase, in that I was now worrying about what might happen if I did kill someone and I had to leave my wife and child behind when I was finally convicted and sent to prison. What would my daughter think, growing up knowing her daddy was a killer? Would I lose them both forever?

For a couple of years such thoughts came and went. I didn't discuss them with Alissa; there seemed little point burdening her with it because I had so many strategies worked out to cope with it. Besides, we were going up in the world. I'd now secured a new job at a solicitors' firm and was doing well. We had more disposable income and we talked about having another child. But when I'm at my happiest I'm often at my most vulnerable with my OCD and anxiety.

I was frightened of losing this happiness and that fear started to send the anxiety into another tailspin.

I became conscious that the handcuffs I still carried around had a key, and that if I did need them to be locked up to prevent harming someone, I could easily unlock them, thereby releasing me from restraint. This preyed on my mind, and very soon the OCD and anxiety was sitting firmly back on my shoulder. I began to wake up feeling depressed, and even wondered if there was any way I could have my arms amputated to make sure I never strangled anyone. Again, it sounds ridiculous here on paper, but these thoughts were very real and were intruding constantly into my everyday life.

Unbeknown to Alissa, I bought 'rescue remedies', herbal tablets, calming pills; anything to take away the anxiety. These didn't seem to work at all, but relief was just over the horizon in the shape of a vacation to Lanzarote, with Alissa's parents. There was packing to be done, things to be purchased, passports to be found. For a few weeks I had a natural distraction and a break to look forward to. Every time the OCD tried to come into my mind, I purposely thought of a positive part of the vacation I was looking forward to, or I distracted myself with planning the vacation. I managed to convince myself that the thoughts running around my mind were just a blip and I could get back to the positive place I was in when I first met and fell in love with Alissa.

Some hope. In the car on the way to the airport, the anxiety which had subsided over the thought of killing someone reappeared in a new form. This time it was asking me a series of insidious questions, over and over again:

'What will you do to take your mind off me?'

'When you stop thinking about me, that's when I'll come back, and what will you do then?'

'You won't forget me. How can you forget me?'

The OCD and anxiety was at full pelt and it was all I could do to drive the car in a straight line. I felt sick with fear. Alissa looked at me, and instinctively knew something was wrong.

'Are you alright, Adam?' she asked. 'You're very quiet ...'

'Oh, it's nothing,' I replied, trying not to crack. 'I've just got a headache, that's all. It'll be alright when we get on the plane.'

We arrived at Manchester Airport and met Alissa's parents at a nearby restaurant. Everyone was meant to be happy. We were supposed to be going on a magical vacation in a lovely villa and all I could think about was the damage my runaway thoughts were doing to me. I don't know how I got on the plane without simply running back through the barrier and out of the airport, but somehow I managed.

All through the flight I held it in, feeling like I was going to explode with pent-up anxiety. We landed, collected our luggage and took a taxi to the villa. Once in our room, I could stand no more. I stood there and just burst into floods of tears. Alissa came running out of the bathroom.

'Adam! What's wrong?! What the hell is wrong?!'

Through my sobs I said that I had something to tell her. Alissa's face darkened. She thought I was about to confess to an affair. If only it were that simple ... I sat her down and explained that I'd had thoughts about bad things happening to people, and that I was scared of losing her, and losing our daughter, and so on.

'Oh, Adam,' she said, 'everyone has thoughts. It doesn't mean because you think something that it's going to happen, you know.'

I couldn't say that I was having thoughts about killing people. I just couldn't do it. What would she think of me, her partner and the father of her child? The man who wanted other children with her? And no matter how much she tried to reassure me, my mind would not let me accept that what I was thinking was indeed 'just a thought'.

Lauren: Adam's actions in buying a set of handcuffs and carrying them around with him so that he wouldn't harm anyone might indeed seem 'bizarre' (as he says) but at the time, he saw it as a logical, responsible action to combat a very disturbing thought.

We describe such an action as a **compulsion, 'safe' behaviour** or a **ritual**. People with OCD seek comfort in compulsions, 'safe' behaviours and rituals because they see them as safety valves for the catastrophic meanings attached to their intrusive thoughts. As we've seen they can be both physical (*'If I carry these handcuffs around I won't kill anyone'*) or mental (*'If I concentrate on all the planning for our vacation my bad thoughts will disappear'* and *'Every time I have a "bad" thought, I will replace it with a "good" and "safe" thought about the vacation.'*) In Adam's case, he was carrying out a compulsion in that he had a 'safety' plan should he suddenly become dangerous (i.e. his handcuffs were in his pocket) so nothing bad would happen. He was also caught up in a **mental avoidance** ritual, in that his 'positive' attitude to planning for a vacation helped to put aside the 'bad' thoughts swirling around his brain. Adam was also doing something we call **neutralising** – he was trying to undo or cancel out the distressing thoughts with ones he thought were positive or safe. Collectively we can call these '**safety behaviours**' because they are actions that OCD and anxiety sufferers carry out to feel safe from their worries.

So let's look at a few examples of obsessions and the compulsions that OCD sufferers use to deal with them:

- (**Obsession**) I have an urge to run across a busy road; therefore, I am a danger to myself and other drivers
- (**Compulsion**) Checking again and again to make sure the road is clear, or avoiding busy roads completely

---

- (**Obsession**) The person who last used this public toilet might have had an incurable disease and I might catch it by using this toilet
- (**Compulsion**) Wiping down every inch of this toilet before I use it, or not using it at all

- (**Obsession**) My father might die on the way to work
- (**Compulsion**) Counting in multiples of three until I 'feel' that this is not going to happen

---

- (**Obsession**) God will punish me for having these impure thoughts
- (**Compulsion**) Praying immediately after an impure thought and undoing the thought by thinking of the charitable work I have done for others

---

- (**Obsession**) My hands are dirty
- (**Compulsion**) Cleaning them until they 'feel' clean (and 'just right')

- (**Obsession**) I have thoughts about harming my newborn child
- (**Compulsion**) I will avoid feeding, bathing, changing my child and let my partner do it so that I do not cause any harm

As we saw in the previous chapter, the **'catastrophic meaning'** of the thought has already been attached, so the next step is for the OCD sufferer to believe they need to take **responsibility** for the thought by doing a compulsion 'safe' behaviour or ritual to neutralise it or make it safe. In Adam's case we can see he is engaging in safety behaviours like buying the handcuffs or avoiding people. Avoidance is vital, and most people with OCD or anxiety problems engage in some kind of avoidance behaviour, i.e. not looking at upsetting images, keeping away from people they feel they might hurt, not going into public toilets, not having knives or other sharp objects around, etc.

As we saw with obsessions and intrusive thoughts, everyone has compulsions to some extent. How many people do you know who deliberately walk under a ladder, just because it's there, or choose Friday 13th to do something risky? Superstition and what has been described as **'magical thinking'** is common among human beings; we all attach some element of 'luck' to things, even if we don't truly believe in it. Why else would you use the same Lottery numbers, year upon year, without winning a penny? The OCD sufferer, on the other hand, believes wholeheartedly in such compulsions and rituals, to the extent that not performing them will most likely result in something catastrophic happening to them and the people around them.

'But,' you might say, 'What's the harm in carrying out a little ritual in order to feel better about something? If it stops you feeling bad, so what?' Well, there is some truth in that – at least at the beginning. If you're anxious about a distressing thought, it's only human nature to try to neutralise, avoid or make amends for that thought. But that means you're taking the thought to be true, or at least very likely to happen, and feeling responsible for stopping or reducing the likely harm – particularly if it involves some kind of unpleasantness – and this can lead to increased anxiety. In fact, because you have to do a compulsion or ritual, you are giving the catastrophic meaning fuel – as you are telling yourself that it is so likely to be true that you have to act! This leads to increased anxiety and self-doubt which can then lead to the OCD sufferer carrying out the compulsion to reduce the perceived harm over and over again and to make sure they have done it properly, as they start distrusting themselves. For example, we've all had the experience where we've left the house and then wondered if we've left an electrical appliance on. You might go back once, just to make sure you didn't. That's an inconvenience, nothing more. But if you check it once, you might walk away and **doubt** that you checked it properly, thus returning to check it again, and then walking away and doubting yourself again and so on. Ironically, even though you are checking the appliance to be sure that you have turned it off, the more you check the appliance, the more you end up doubting yourself that you have actually turned it off!

There is also the element of **seeking reassurance**. We will look at this in more depth later on but in short, it's when sufferers reassure themselves, in a variety of ways, that bad things won't happen and they will not carry out the action they most worry about. It can take the form of asking repeated questions ('Am I mad?' 'Have you touched anything dirty at work?') or, increasingly now, by searching the internet for various subjects or issues. The problem with reassurance is threefold; for a start, it reinforces the fear that something is bad or wrong. Secondly, your anxiety problem is very clever and reassurance will never ever be enough – it will keep needing more and more reassurance. Thirdly, especially when on the internet, you almost always find something that confirms your fears, however wrong it is, which will only make you worry even more!

So carrying out compulsions and rituals becomes counter-productive. It might bring relief at first, but the more complicated and/or frequent the ritual becomes, the more it reinforces the strength of the initial obsession, bringing increasing anxiety and disturbance to everyday life. Adam's anxiety increased to the extent that he was taking all sorts of pills and potions to prevent it – in fact, without realising he was simply fuelling it. He didn't stop to think what might happen if he DIDN'T do any of his rituals or threw his handcuffs in the bin. By then, it was too late.

Adam had attached a catastrophic meaning to his thoughts, taken responsibility for preventing harm, engaged in compulsions or rituals (safety behaviours) to reduce the perceived likelihood of the harm occurring and therefore increased his anxiety and self-doubt.

In short, he treated the thought with the seriousness **it did not deserve in the first place**.

Had he not done so, and not engaged in rituals, and simply accepted the thought for what it was – just a thought – what would have happened? Would he really have strangled someone? Of course not, but the belief and conviction he had in the worrying thought was enough to convince him otherwise.

So safety behaviours actually reinforce the message of danger. Adam bought the handcuffs and said, 'Now I don't have to worry any more,' but actually he was saying 'I know I'm dangerous but now I have handcuffs I won't do anything.' He was reinforcing the message that something was wrong with him and that he was liable to be dangerous.

In addition, a safety behaviour can mutate and no matter what you do, it will never be 'enough' to keep you safe. Adam eventually realised that because he had the handcuff keys he could simply unlock himself and do the harm to others he believed he would do. He was constantly asking himself '**What if?**' – a very common phrase among OCD and anxiety sufferers. 'What if I throw away the key?' 'What if I find it again?' 'What if I unlock myself?' and so on. This leads on to rumination – a mental behaviour that attempts to deal with upsetting thoughts by thinking about them over and over again in the hope they will finally be solved. When Adam was thinking about the handcuffs he was both employing the 'What if?' scenario and ruminating on his thoughts, which then gets stuck on an unhelpful mental loop. OCD sufferers then start to question whether they are, in fact, mad, and will be locked up because they've actually gone insane. Their OCD has now mutated into a new form and has become about going insane. Sufferers will start to search the internet about mental illness and will become terrified at anyone finding out that they're having such thoughts, in case the police or psychiatrists are called and they are taken away. This is very serious, because although they are not mad, OCD can actually stop people seeking the very help they need. They will feel ashamed that they're having such thoughts, and will again not dare to seek help. If this is you, please do not worry – you are NOT mad, you are NOT alone, and you should never be ashamed to seek help.

Stopping seeking help can also apply to people having intrusive thoughts about their children, as Adam had, or children you spend time with. These thoughts are common, and also very distressing. Although Adam's thoughts didn't attach to his daughter directly, we must remember that OCD can attach itself to anything, including the people and things we care about the most.

Types of intrusions that people may have around their own children or children they spend time with are that they might harm the child in some way, including abusing them. Other common worries are that they might pass on their illness to the children or that they are bad parents for having unpleasant intrusive thoughts. Some examples of common catastrophic meanings that parents and other caregivers attach to these intrusions include:

- 'I am dangerous around (my) children, and therefore need to stay away from them.'
- 'I can't be trusted around children and I need to be supervised if I have contact with them.'
- 'It must mean I am a paedophile therefore I cannot be around children.'
- 'These thoughts mean I don't love my children and am a bad parent who doesn't deserve to have children.'

- 'If I tell anyone about my thoughts, then my children will be removed from my care.'

This last thought is a very common worry in OCD; that Social Services will take the children away if parents or caregivers disclose their thoughts. This becomes a barrier for people seeking help because they worry that if anyone knows about these thoughts, they will assume they are dangerous and not fit parents and will report them to Social Services. As with the thoughts of going mad, people with worries around children will invariably research this on the internet as a compulsion, and as you will know, researching the problem will only find evidence confirming that this has happened – that the medical practitioner has misunderstood OCD and alerted Social Services, who in turn do not understand OCD and decided that the sufferer was dangerous to their children, and subsequently removed the children.

Unfortunately, this has happened but only in very, very rare circumstances. And medical practitioners are now much more aware of mental health problems, including OCD, so are likely to recommend you see a psychiatrist or psychologist first. If you are worried about this happening, and it is stopping you from seeking help, then you should seek help from a psychologist or psychiatrist experienced in anxiety problems, or seek advice from one of the OCD or mental health charities who can help guide you on the best course of action to getting help. For further information or support, please visit our global charity organisation at www.shawmindfoundation.org. In the PTT approach in Part II of this book we will also give you some very useful strategies to deal with intrusive thoughts around children.

CHAPTER 5

BREAKING DOWN AND TELLING ALL

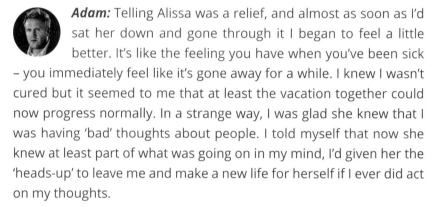 *Adam:* Telling Alissa was a relief, and almost as soon as I'd sat her down and gone through it I began to feel a little better. It's like the feeling you have when you've been sick – you immediately feel like it's gone away for a while. I knew I wasn't cured but it seemed to me that at least the vacation together could now progress normally. In a strange way, I was glad she knew that I was having 'bad' thoughts about people. I told myself that now she knew at least part of what was going on in my mind, I'd given her the 'heads-up' to leave me and make a new life for herself if I ever did act on my thoughts.

We went for a meal that evening and as we walked back to the villa we passed a bookstall. I wanted something to read, so I picked up an autobiography by Ronnie O'Sullivan, the British world champion snooker player. The back cover mentioned his battle with depression, so I bought it. I knew I was suffering from an element of depression connected with whatever was going on in my head but, being a generally positive person, I couldn't really understand where it was coming from. I hoped the book might have the answers.

Over the next few days I became absorbed by Ronnie's story and felt we had something in common. It inspired me to make the decision that I would take exercise and get fit, as Ronnie did during his bouts of depression. I started jogging the day after. I guess that was a safety behaviour to take my mind away from my worries, but there is positivity in exercise and whenever I had a troubling thought I'd go back to Ronnie's book or take off for a run.

Flying home from Lanzarote made me realise how much I missed being around aircraft, and how sorry I was that I wasn't flying the plane myself. I knew I was heading back to work at the solicitors and while it was a good job, there was a part of me that felt something was missing. I longed to create an opportunity for myself which would mean I could be in control of my own destiny. I needed a vocation in life; something that would have me leaping out of bed every morning. The thought nagged at me and I went back to work with a heavy heart.

Predictably, after a couple of weeks my thoughts spiralled out of control again and I hit rock bottom. I couldn't even get out of bed, never mind go to work. I was crying on the phone to my boss, trying to explain in as general terms as possible that I was sick and wouldn't be able to go in. If I raised my head to look out of the bedroom window I'd see people walking past and I'd have thoughts of strangling them. Alissa must have been wondering what on earth she'd hitched herself to …

In short, I had a full-on breakdown. It had been two years since the last episode and I think my parents thought they'd seen the last of my worries, especially now I'd found a lovely partner and become a father. Alissa phoned my mum and told her I was very poorly. My parents sensibly called out the emergency Mental Health team and they responded quickly. I was asked to go for an assessment and, alone with them, I described everything that had gone on; the thoughts of hurting people, the fear around knives, the obsession about stabbing old people and children. Even if they carted me off and threw away the key, they had to know the lot.

Well, they didn't take me away. The two people who assessed me sat very calmly as I explained everything. When I'd finished, the male nurse took a breath then smiled.

'Have you ever heard of OCD, Adam?' he asked.

'Isn't that when people can't stop turning lights on and off?' I asked, remembering doing that myself when I was younger.

'It is,' the nurse said, 'but it's about a lot of other things too.'

'We find that quite a few people with OCD are the ones who care a lot,' the female nurse chipped in, 'because you find something so horrifying you believe you'll end up doing it.'

As I listened, what they were saying started to make sense. For the first time ever, I was getting something of an explanation about my behaviour. I was also hearing that I wasn't a monster or a mass murderer. I was an ordinary person with thoughts that had become out of control, driven by an overload of fear. I did worry a lot and I did have repetitive behaviour. Everything they said seemed to tick another box. They recommended I see a doctor, and that I needed a course of Cognitive Behavioural Therapy (CBT). I had no idea what that was and so it was explained to me that it was a way of looking at thought patterns that would help me understand and see them for what they were.

They weren't experts but the mental health nurses gave me hope: hope that I would be able to one day control my thoughts and lift myself out of chronic anxiety and depression. I was referred quite quickly and within a week I was sitting in front of a specialist psychiatrist who would either confirm the OCD diagnosis or offer his own explanation.

Alissa came with me and, for the first time, heard the full story. I was terribly nervous about her listening to all this, but she took it in her stride. If she was worried she didn't show it. The doctor was somewhat impersonal but he carried out the checks and tests very comprehensively. He asked me if I heard voices or had hallucinations. I didn't.

'Then I'm pretty sure it's OCD, as you've been told,' he said.

He told me I could go on medication straight away, which would be Fluoxetine, an antidepressant used to treat OCD. In addition, I would be placed on a waiting list for CBT which, under the National Health Service in the UK, would mean that it would be around six months before I could start treatment. Luckily for me, my parents offered to pay for an immediate course of private treatment, and so towards the end of this awful episode of my life I started out with my first therapist, based in Sheffield.

Lauren: Firstly, let's look at a couple of things going on with Adam in this chapter. It's clear that just before he arrived in Lanzarote, and while he was there, he suffered from acute panic attacks brought on by a heightened level of anxiety, worrying that his obsessions and compulsions were out of control.

We mentioned in the previous chapter that relying on compulsions or rituals to negate or avoid obsessions or intrusive thoughts is, in the long term, a most unhelpful response. Instead of pushing the intrusion away, they actually make it stronger, creating a kind of whirlpool of anxiety which begins to spin faster and faster. Adam's fears about harming people became out of control on the way to the airport, resulting in a near-nervous breakdown. Telling Alissa what was going on helped, but back in England he again suffered the sensation of his thoughts spiralling out of control, sending him crashing down once more.

Anxiety goes hand-in-hand with OCD, for the reasons I've explained above, and is a normal response to stress or danger. Anxiety is better known as the body's **'fight, flight or freeze'** mechanism; you either stand your ground against the thing that is threatening you, or you run away from it, or in some cases you freeze or play 'dead'. These actions are designed to keep you as safe as possible – an inbuilt survival mechanism. Adrenalin is pumped through your system quickly, enabling you to make that snap decision – do I stay, do I run or do I freeze? As I've said, it's a normal response, and it only becomes a problem when it either misfires (that the threat is not real or disproportionate to the actual scenario) or you experience it in relation to a very unlikely threat (such as killing someone, in Adam's case).

> **Anxiety is not trying to hurt you. It is trying to do its job and protect you.**

For example, Adam has not yet realised that his thought about harming people is just that: only a thought. So his response has been to take responsibility for it, and go out of his way to stop himself from carrying out that thought. As the thought has taken hold (because he's given it a catastrophic meaning) his response to it becomes out of proportion and so his 'fight, flight or freeze' mechanism kicks in strongly, causing heightened anxiety. In some cases this can lead to panic attacks.

Panic attacks are by no means uncommon among OCD and anxiety sufferers. Indeed, if you feel you have OCD and you're reading this, just the words 'panic attack' may already be triggering feelings of heightened anxiety. This isn't surprising, as panic attacks are frightening and, if you haven't had one before, they can appear to come out of nowhere. You feel like you've been given something toxic, like a psychedelic drug, and you feel you have no control over your thoughts, emotions and sometimes even your physical actions. For the OCD and anxiety sufferer they seem to reinforce the 'seriousness' of the thought pattern that has led you to the attack in the first place. You feel something awful is about to happen to you.

However, if you have read this far and understood everything I've said about obsessions, intrusions, catastrophic meanings and rituals/compulsions and safety behaviours, you will know that OCD has only attached itself to your thoughts. If you have a panic attack, please try to remember that it is just a heightened reaction to a normal bodily process; be mindful of what is happening to you, acknowledge it is really unpleasant, but understand that it is just a normal although intense anxiety reaction.

Part II of this book will show you a simple way of dealing with and recovering from panic attacks. We will examine practical ways of coping with panic attacks so that you will not feel overwhelmed if and when they occur. Above all, we will teach you not to associate places, people or events with panic attacks, which may otherwise cause you to avoid situations or places that you think may trigger such attacks.

Adam's arrival back in the UK coincides with another crash, in which he says 'he couldn't get out of bed' and had 'hit rock bottom'. He is still having intrusive thoughts about harming people, and the panic and anxiety is obviously affecting him significantly. In addition, his mood is low; he cannot motivate himself to go to work (or do anything at all) and is spending a significant amount of time in tears.

In short, Adam is also suffering from depression. It's hardly surprising, given what he's going through at this stage and the fact that his compulsions and rituals to control his OCD don't appear to be working any more. OCD is ruling his life, and restricting it to such an extent that I'd be surprised if anyone in his state of mind wasn't depressed. How could you not be?

We'll look at depression a little later in our recovery approach in Part II. For now, let me just say that it is important to be clear that **Adam's depression is a result of his OCD, and not the other way round**.

When I first met Adam I was of the opinion that he was depressed, but only because of the impact the OCD was having on his life. He did not suffer from depression before the OCD, and had periods of managing the OCD without depression. It's important to make the distinction, because **if your depression pre-dates your OCD, or is so serious that it prevents you from being able to engage in the help you need to beat the anxiety or OCD problem, the depression side needs to be treated as a separate entity** (please visit www.shawmindfoundation.org for further information on depression). A therapist will be able to treat you for the OCD and anxiety, but the depression might need to be examined on its own. However, if your depression is a result of your OCD and it doesn't pre-date your OCD symptoms, and it is not a barrier to getting well, then a therapist will focus on the OCD first. Once that is being managed, a reduction in the symptoms of depression, such as Adam was having above, will almost certainly occur.

Also in this chapter we saw Adam telling Alissa about his obsessions and compulsions, then letting everything out – including the fears of harming other people – to the Mental Health team during his assessment.

So when should you tell those around you that you're suffering from OCD or an anxiety problem (or at least, you feel something is wrong and you have acute anxiety episodes or OCD-like symptoms)? Well, it could be that they'll already know something isn't right and just haven't mentioned it, for fear of upsetting you. If you've been avoiding people, places and things, or you've been asking the same question of them over and over again, or you've tried to make them follow your obsessional rules, the chances are they have noticed that you're behaving oddly. It's quite often the case that people around an OCD sufferer know something is amiss even before the sufferer themselves. You're so busy trying to keep yourself and others safe from your thoughts, or avoiding them altogether, that you're not looking externally at yourself and the changes in your behaviour. And because your compulsions and rituals are becoming more frequent and complex, you have less time for those around you. However, in the case of people suffering from other anxiety problems, it is not always clear to others that they have a problem. They have usually become so expert at hiding it, or avoiding things that they believe may trigger the anxiety.

With OCD, you might be unconsciously alerting people to your difficulties via 'reassurance' behaviour, which we talked about in the last chapter. That is, you're constantly asking those around you to double-check that doors are locked and the cooker is off (if your obsessions are around checking), or whether they have cleaned their shoes properly before coming inside or if they have washed their hands (if you have obsessions around contamination), or you may be constantly seeking the opinion that you're not, after all, a 'bad' person.

That said, sharing the problem in a way that makes others understand what you are going through is extremely helpful and, as Adam demonstrates, is very often the first step to breaking the cycle of OCD, anxiety and related depression. Of course, this very much depends on you, the sufferer, having an understanding of your problem and it may be that even though you've read this far you're still wondering: does any of this relate to me? In Part II of the book we will look at ways you can self-diagnose and begin to understand all the elements of OCD and anxiety as they apply to you personally, and it might only be then that you feel confident enough to share your problem.

If you feel ready now to make a disclosure, then it could be really helpful for the person you are about to disclose to, to read this book as well! They will then have a better insight into anxiety, obsessions, intrusions, catastrophic meanings, compulsions, rituals etc. and you will then feel more able to share and discuss what's going on for you.

You need to be able to transmit the fact that although having OCD and anxiety is not your fault, it can become a powerful force when people (like you) are stuck with thoughts that make them anxious and make them act in certain ways. These actions are not scary, but in fact are motivated by the prevention of harm, avoidance of a dangerous situation, or a desire to banish the thoughts. You can also point out that while you feel the need to seek reassurance, it isn't that helpful to receive it.

So as an exercise, next time you seek reassurance from your partner, family member or friend that they have checked the locks/ the gas cooker/the iron or washed their hands or that you are not a dangerous person etc., try to remember that it's just OCD – a thought, nothing more. Remind yourself, **reassurance is a short-term strategy that will make the OCD and self-doubt worse in the long run**. Don't ask for it, and see what happens.

I should add that you *may* find the person you disclose to doesn't understand, and reacts in a way which is counter-productive. **If this happens, please don't worry**. Not everyone is psychologically equipped to understand what's going on for you and it may be fearful for some people, particularly those close to you, to think that you're having troublesome thoughts. If this is the case, then don't hide away; make an appointment to see a medical practitioner, psychiatrist or psychologist, explain to them how you're feeling and bring this book along to share with the doctor. The medical practitioner might not be a specialist but will have empathy and understanding, and will be able to refer you to the right people.

CHAPTER 6

'JUST FEAR'

Adam: Working with my first-ever therapist, Michael, was the first time that I began to explore the implications of OCD and anxiety. This investigation itself gave me some comfort; previously, I'd thought I was a psychopath or a potential mass murderer. Having a name for what I was going through and knowing that I wasn't alone was a real help at a time when, up to this point, all I'd done was run away from whatever was troubling me.

The real 'lightbulb' moment came, however, when Michael put into one sentence what I was experiencing.

'The sensations you're having, Adam,' he said, 'are just fear. Not reality – just fear.'

Just fear. Those two words struck me like a bullet between the eyes. At that moment, I saw my condition for what it was. I wasn't some crazed axe murderer having voices telling me what to do. This was simply a sensation of fear that I would carry out the acts that were rolling around my mind – nothing more, nothing less.

'You will not do these things, Adam,' said Michael, 'It's just fear Believe me.'

I did, and for the first time I'd seen a qualified professional therapist who was able to define what I was going through and give a plausible explanation for it. Naturally, I was on a high.

'It's just fear,' I told myself, 'Just fear. I'm fine.'

Suddenly I had the answer and I assumed that I was cured. I carried on seeing Michael for a couple more weeks, but now I was confident I knew what it was, I was keen to put it behind me and get on with my life.

Michael suggested I carried on with him. 'No thanks,' I said, 'I'm done. I'm cured.' And so I left, and at the same time I took myself off the Fluoxetine medication I'd been prescribed by the doctor. What was the point of carrying on with those now I was fixed? Besides, my parents had been paying for the therapy and I didn't want to financially burden them for longer than I needed to.

However, I didn't leave with any kind of technique or true understanding of how to deal with this fear; I had no foundations on which to build my recovery. What I needed to learn was how to **accept** and **embrace** the fear; not to question it but to take it on board, in all its horrible glory. Instead, I ran away, convinced I had the solution. I wanted to make the bad thoughts disappear, and now I had the method. Whenever I had a disturbing thought, all I needed to tell myself was that 'it is just fear' until it made me feel right. Easy.

The problem was that by telling myself over and over again that it was 'just fear', I was creating a method of distraction that would itself become a ritual I needed as part of my everyday life. The anxiety hadn't gone away, but I could dissipate it with the repetition of the 'just fear' phrase. Predictably, communicating this mantra to myself became important for the recovery I thought I was having.

That said, I did feel better, and seemed to be in a place where I could start to make some life-changing decisions. Having messed up my flying career, I needed a new challenge that would allow me to be my own boss. OCD or not, I've always been good at generating ideas and putting strategies in place to make things happen. I didn't purposely harness my OCD and anxiety but I did have a lot of energy and adrenalin, possibly fuelled by the fear that my OCD could come back at any time and overwhelm me. Although I didn't know it, I was still controlled by my anxiety, but oddly it was this which drove the desire in me to be the best.

I found the outlet for all this within my job at the solicitors. The firm was representing former coal miners who were suffering, or had suffered from, severe respiratory illnesses, along with their families. We were bringing claims against the British government's Department of Trade and Industry and while we were winning large sums of money, some of it wasn't going to the right family members simply because many miners hadn't made a last will and testament.

I suggested that we should offer will-writing and estate planning as part of our service, but the senior partners didn't seem interested.

The idea nagged at me, and I found out that you didn't need to be a qualified solicitor to write wills for other people. However, you did need training and so I went on a course and learned how to do it. I thought that if I could offer a bespoke will-writing service as part of a package for financial advisers to sell to their clients, I might pick up customers quickly.

I left my job, bought a PC from a chainstore and worked from my bedroom. I was determined that my service would outstrip any competition; looking better, offering more, being the best on the market. I had a website designed and networked financial advisers as hard as I could. Within three or four months I was pulling in clients, writing wills and making an income that previously I could have only dreamt about. The next stage was to offer a service to financial advisers whereby they could learn how to write wills themselves. My business grew exponentially again, especially after the global financial crash of 2008 when financial advisers were desperately looking to survive and diversify following the drying up of the mortgage market.

The setting up of my business in 2006 also coincided with another important event, for just two days before I launched the company Alissa gave birth to our second daughter. Unlike our first daughter's birth, I had no concerns around thoughts of harming this child because now I had the 'just fear' phrase I could employ whenever I felt a thought was getting out of control. During her birth, I did have a thought around strangling a doctor, who wouldn't then be able to deliver any more babies, bringing chaos into the lives of other pregnant women, but I was able to dismiss this quickly with 'just fear' – the magic phrase.

Quickly, my business became very successful and, driven by OCD and anxiety, I was working harder and harder to sustain my success and build a solid foundation for my company. After a few years we moved from the three-bedroom semi-detached house we'd been living in and put our children in private school. I even treated myself to an Aston Martin DB9. I believe it's human nature to want to aspire and move up in the world, and I wanted us all to enjoy the benefits of my newfound wealth.

Building the business served as an effective distraction from OCD and anxiety. And I could still do my rituals and no one would suspect what was going on in my head. Of course, I couldn't tell anyone about that. It would have attracted incredible stigma, and to this day, none of my business colleagues and employees know what I've been through. So I went to some lengths to disguise it, even to the point that I would mock people with depression, saying they didn't have the energy and enthusiasm to thrive in a business environment. I'm not proud to say I acted like that. I was ashamed about the thoughts in my head, so I took great pains not to show any perceived weakness.

I wasn't the best boss at that time. I was a ruthless dictator, wanting to control absolutely everything and everybody. When it's your money you're risking you want it your way, and you believe no one can be as good or committed as you. Now I've accepted and embraced my OCD through to recovery, I hope I'm a much better person to work for and a far better businessman for it.

Although my drive was, and still is, based around wanting to provide for my family, I wasn't easy to live with during this period. Everything was focused around the business, and Alissa and the kids didn't get much of a look in. By this stage, 2010, our next daughter had arrived on the scene and so we had three young children around the house. I was working harder and harder, and pushing my 'bad' thoughts aside by using the 'just fear' mantra, up to thirty times a day if I was having a particularly bad episode.

If anything went wrong at work it would be reflected at home, and I wasn't as respectful of Alissa as I should've been. Young ambitious males can also be very selfish, and I was no exception. Luckily, Alissa was rather more mature than me and took everything in her stride. I loved the kids and did try with them, but they weren't the distraction for me that business was. I needed to be buzzing with work, and that was what drove me on. Besides, the 'just fear' mantra was becoming tiring, and there were occasions it didn't seem to work. I found it particularly hard to be around sharp knives, and if one of the kids asked me to cut them a slice of bread or peel an apple I'd make an excuse not to do it. They probably thought I was being lazy but I couldn't face having a sharp kitchen knife in my hands, near the kids.

Did I ever have intrusive thoughts in other situations involving the kids, particularly when we were in vulnerable situations? The answer is yes, but again it wasn't so much *about* the kids as *around* them. Sometimes when we were in the car, and the kids were in the back, I'd have a thought that I'd suddenly accelerate at a crossing and run over the pedestrian in front of me. To counter that, I'd slow down at the crossing just like any other driver, and then I'd press the brake really hard, as though I was forcing the bad thought away through the pedal. That would relieve the stress around the thought and I'd be able to continue driving normally. Despite such thoughts I never stopped driving, thinking that if I had a really bad episode of anxiety I'd be able to pull over and let Alissa drive. People with OCD and anxiety excel at hiding things, and using the brake technique to dispel a thought is a perfect example. For all anyone knew we were just on another car journey, not intending to harm anyone.

Alissa put up with a hell of a lot and it's only now that I can repay her for those years. Today, I'm a lot more relaxed around the kids and I hope I'm a good husband. Certainly, I'm more mature than I was, and have learned to be happy about my success in business, which is closely aligned with the techniques and approach to OCD and life post-recovery that Lauren introduced me to, found in Part II of this book.

Could I have built up the business without OCD and anxiety? I often ask myself that question and the honest answer is that I just don't know. OCD is part of my make-up, part of my life, and our characteristics and genetic inheritance make us all follow the paths we do. If I hadn't had OCD I would perhaps have chosen a different path, but while my OCD has been horrendous it has helped to take me to where I'm very pleased to be now. Sometimes you need the bad times to make the good times better. Perhaps I'd have been a qualified pilot now, but OCD and anxiety stopped me doing that and I followed a different path. Again, sometimes it's the parts of us we don't like that actually open the doors for us.

Sadly, the door opening for me, even as the business was becoming more successful, was one that led to a very dark place. Five years had now passed since my last appointment with my private therapist, Michael. So many changes had happened in my life during this period and my anxiety was increasing, based on the perception that I could lose everything at any time, and fuelled by the notion that the 'only fear' ritual was no longer working. I kept repeating the phrase over and over again, but now my mind was asking the questions: 'What if this doesn't work? What if my therapist was wrong? What will happen then? Will everything fall apart?' I was about to be pitched into a darkness that would overwhelm me and almost drive me to the point of no return.

 Lauren: As we discussed towards the end of the last chapter, Adam has done absolutely the right thing in seeking help from medical professionals and a therapist. Learning that he has OCD is a huge relief for him, particularly when he realises he is by no means alone. According to statistics, OCD could affect as many as 1–2 in every 100 people (1–2 per cent of the population) right across age, gender and background.[5] The World Health Organisation (WHO[6]) has actually ranked OCD in the top ten of the most disabling illnesses of any kind, in terms of lost earnings and diminished quality of life. So Adam is not alone, and neither are you.

However, this is not the end of Adam's story. The important element in this chapter is about his attempts to 'fix' his OCD with his first therapist and how that became a ritual in itself.

If you've read this far you'll understand that while OCD can have simple beginnings, it can also be incredibly tricky and complex at times. That doesn't mean we can't overcome it ourselves if we try, but we must be aware of its complexity. If you don't follow the right method of treatment for OCD and anxiety, the OCD will let you think you're on top of it – but in fact, it will simply reinforce it.

As an example, let's look at the message which was given to Adam about his OCD being 'just fear'. His first therapist was correct to tell Adam this, as OCD is certainly a fear-based disorder. However, what doesn't seem to have been explained to Adam is that the fear (or as I'd call it, **the thought**) has to have a **catastrophic meaning** attached to it, which is the **trigger** for the **compulsion** to develop, and turn into OCD.

---

5 American Psychiatric Association. (2013). *Diagnostic and Statistical Manual of Mental Disorders* (5th ed.). Arlington, VA: American Psychiatric Publishing.
6 The World Health Organisation http://www.who.int/en/.

Let's go right back to the beginning. You're walking over a bridge and you suddenly have an **intrusive thought** about jumping into the water. Let's say you attach a **catastrophic meaning** to it (*'I've just thought about jumping into the river. It must mean I'm suicidal and something is very wrong with me and I can't be left on my own because I'm likely to cause harm to myself.'*) This is the trigger for compulsions, which might include: avoiding bridges, high places, busy roads, knives or anything that might be used as a means of suicide; surrounding yourself constantly by family or friends to keep an eye on you so you don't lose control and commit suicide; and researching all types of mental illness to try and find out what is wrong with you and what treatment you need, such as a secure facility to keep you locked up and safe.

So yes, it is 'just fear' but we don't properly understand why it's just fear until we've had the process explained to us. And because Adam hadn't had that sequence outlined to him, and therefore never had the opportunity of challenging the meaning of what he was thinking, he took up the phrase 'just fear' as a mantra to protect himself.

And in doing so, he created another ritual or safety behaviour which reinforced his OCD.

I don't blame him for this. By now, you'll understand the pain and suffering Adam had been through to get to the stage where he sought help. All he wanted was to feel better and for his OCD to go away and leave him alone. And *'just fear'* worked for a while, until **'What if...?'** started to creep in and cast doubt on the strength of the comfort blanket he was grasping on to.

The way to differentiate between rituals and strategies to overcome OCD that will work in the long term is to ask: 'What is the purpose of this? Is it making me feel better at the moment? Does it reduce my anxiety immediately and do I feel reassured that the feared outcome will not happen right now?' If you find that whatever you're doing or saying to yourself reduces your anxiety immediately, and you feel relieved that the disastrous outcome is delayed for now, it's probably more of a ritual than a long-term strategy, and in the long term it's not going to be helpful.

Part of the treatment for OCD and anxiety which we will look at in depth in our recovery approach located in Part II of this book, is that **sufferers have to face their fears and experience anxiety** in order to get through it. By facing fear and experiencing anxiety – pulling the trigger on our thoughts and the meanings they have for us – we come to understand the obsessions, catastrophic meanings and compulsions around our OCD or anxiety and only then can we become fully aware that, in fact, what we're facing is indeed 'just fear'. It's by no means an easy path but it is the only one to take if you're serious about overcoming OCD and anxiety, and living a life free of it.

Before we move towards the application of our PTT treatment approach, let me reiterate something we touched upon in Chapter 4, that of anxiety-related worries centering on children. A common problem in OCD occurs when someone is pregnant or has recently given birth, and while we see that Adam's thoughts haven't attached themselves to his new baby, he does have obsessions around what is going on in the delivery room. Not only is being pregnant and giving birth a frequently overwhelming situation for both men, and especially for women, who experience incredible hormonal changes, but it alters life for both parents. Suddenly they are solely responsible for this tiny helpless baby. It is very common for people to have intrusive thoughts which might include 'What if I smother my baby accidentally?' or 'What if I drowned my baby in the bath?' or 'What if I throw the baby down the stairs?' How scary for a new parent to have these thoughts!

I can assure you, OCD or no OCD, every new parent has these thoughts.

Uncomfortable as they are, they are normal and they are just thoughts, and understandable in the context of being a new parent. However, people both with a history of OCD or no previous OCD have gone on to develop OCD in these circumstances. In fact, there is growing awareness that this is an important time to offer support to new parents if they have a history of OCD or have developed OCD. Please visit www.shawmindfoundation.org for information on Maternal OCD and support to help mothers with OCD (both perinatal and postnatal). We will also look at strategies to deal with such thoughts in the PTT treatment approach in Part II of this book.

Adam's account alludes to OCD being something of a 'positive' force in his life. He accepts that OCD has been part of his life, and in some way has 'helped' to give him the drive he needed to be a success. He is confident about saying this now, because he understands his OCD and how to deal with it. You, as a reader, might wonder why he's accepted a condition so harrowing into his life. The fact is, accepting and embracing OCD as a part of him has given him the tools to be able to control it. He sees the positives in it – but is that just because he is who he is? Is it the same for everyone? Can we all see positives in our OCD?

As we know, OCD is a mental disorder and it has to be significantly interfering in your life in order to be diagnosed as such. However, there are often aspects of OCD-type thinking or responding that may have a positive effect on a person's life. For example, we often find people have 'all-or-nothing' thinking patterns and this might push them on to become outstanding athletes or successful in business (as Adam is). The British footballer David Beckham has admitted having difficulties with obsessive-compulsive type behaviour, but it hasn't stopped him from being one of the world's most famous players and ambassadors for the game.

Obviously, not everyone with OCD traits goes on to become a famous footballer or successful in business, as our thinking and behaving patterns combine with a lot of other factors. You don't have to be a perfectionist to have OCD, but therapists often find perfectionism and unrelenting high standards among their clients with anxiety. Sometimes that can be helpful and help us strive, achieve and do well, but there is also a maladaptive side of perfectionism. It may be that Adam has a combination of being driven, with high standards and an all-or-nothing thinking style, but this was combined with being naturally bright and determined to be his own boss. In addition, his desire to strive harder and harder could also be avoidance in that the harder he worked, the less attention he paid to unpleasant thoughts or feelings. Usually what we find is that regardless of how successful you've become, if you have OCD or an anxiety problem, it won't go away without proper intervention, and at some point it will come back to interfere in your life.

And if you look at other famous people with OCD and anxiety, you'll see that not all stories end in success. Howard Hughes, the American billionaire and philanthropist, was an incredibly successful and wealthy man, but he ended up living a miserable existence because of his severe OCD. Conversely, it's true that you can have OCD, be very successful and not need treatment for a while, and you can get on well in life. I've met people who've had OCD since they were quite young and it didn't intrude until their mid-to-late-thirties because they managed to keep it under some form of control. You have to think how strong such people are to be coping with a disorder as well as living a life, maintaining relationships and achieving at work. But the important thing to note is: **without your OCD you will still be all these things**. You will still be successful and achieve and maintain relationships and, if anything, life might be better for you because you won't be hampered by the anxiety AND you will still have these positive traits. So please do not think that getting treatment and getting better from OCD and anxiety is in any way going to inhibit your performance or reduce your success. As we shall see, if anything, it will do the opposite.

CHAPTER 7

THE POINT OF NO RETURN?

Adam: I'd spent almost eight years building up a business from a one-man operation in a bedroom to an organisation on a very successful financial footing with hundreds of employees. It was a dream come true, yet I had a nagging sense that things were still not right in my mind. The OCD and anxiety were never far from the surface and had begun to creep in on a more regular basis.

In February 2012 our first son was born. His was a difficult birth; he weighed more than 10 lbs and had to be resuscitated just after he was delivered. That was one of the most stressful hours of our lives. Alissa was crying her eyes out, thinking he was stillborn. Eventually the nurses got him going and he was fine, but it was a terrible episode. I remember distinctly feeling that I was going to cry and because I didn't want to do it in front of Alissa I made an excuse and headed for my car, parked in the hospital car park.

I sat there, and for an hour just wept and wept. It wasn't just about the baby and the awful birth; all the stress around the business, the ups and downs that go with employing people and making a success of things, plus all the 'bad' thoughts swirling around my head caused an outpouring of emotion that I thought would never stop. I felt so tired with everything, particularly the ongoing battle with my OCD and anxiety. After an hour I went back into the hospital and spent ten minutes in the gents' bathroom, washing my face and trying to look normal. Alissa was mad – she'd wondered where I'd wandered off to so soon after such a traumatic episode. I couldn't tell her the truth.

Around this time my company made its first acquisition, which we thought would help expand our services to expatriate British people who had retired to Spain and the surrounding Spanish islands.

As managing director I was spending a lot of time in Lanzarote overseeing the deal and setting up our own operation. The weather was good and I enjoyed the lifestyle, but I missed Alissa and the kids. They loved being in the sun so it made sense for them all to come over and join me. We could rent a villa and be together as a family.

So in 2013, just a year after our first son was born, that's what we did. We've never been a family that has followed preconceived ideas of what we should do and when, and so a temporary move to Lanzarote made complete sense. I'd got to the point where I was financially comfortable and my kids would have the perfect outdoor life in a beautiful, sunny climate. So they all came over and we spent weekends in the pool and had barbecues every evening. People would look at me and tell me that I had 'the dream life'. And it was true. I had no more worries.

But true to form, I began to worry that I had no more worries. In addition, my supposedly carefree lifestyle was leading me into bad habits. I was eating more and exercising less, and quite quickly I reached 18 stone (250 lbs) in weight. I was lazy, lethargic and tired, and I shouldn't have been any of these things because I was free to do what I wanted, when I wanted. Yet I could barely be bothered to take the children to school and whereas at first I would play with them in the pool most evenings, I didn't have the inclination or the energy. Also, I was beginning to feel a little bit depressed.

I should have read the warning signs before it was too late. Instead, I ignored them and carried on with my 'only fear' ritual, which clearly wasn't working any more. More than seven years had now passed since seeing my private therapist, Michael. Once again, I was becoming a prisoner of my OCD and anxiety, and running away from all the tension that was rising inside me.

I will never forget the day the OCD crashed back into me like a tsunami. About a mile from the villa lay a beautiful beach with lagoons dotted around where the kids could fish. We decided to go down there for the afternoon, take a picnic and let the kids enjoy themselves by the water. We had to drive through a short tunnel to get there and just on the other side was a bridge. As we emerged I spotted an old lady standing by the side of it.

'If I wanted, I could pull over now and strangle her, and no one would have the power to stop me,' I thought.

The sensation crept into me like ice through my veins. It had been years since a thought like this had caused me so much distress: there was a poor old lady who I could attack, and no one was strong enough to prevent it, least of all me.

'It's just fear, just fear, just fear,' I told myself desperately. But it didn't work. My OCD and anxiety was now in charge, laughing at me for giving in to it.

We stopped at a supermarket to buy some bottled water. I got out of the car hastily like I was gasping for air. Alissa and the kids stayed in the car. I reached the shop and wandered through the store in a daze. I felt drained, as if I'd lost pints of blood. I couldn't stop thinking about the old lady, and how to get the image of me strangling her out of my head. The more I tried, the more invasive it was. All I wanted to do was enjoy a day out with my wife and kids, but my thoughts wouldn't let me go.

I grabbed a few bottles of water and went to the checkout. A girl sat behind the desk, idly scanning customers' items and taking the money.

'What if these thoughts never let you go?' I said to myself. *'What if you decided to strangle the checkout girl? What would happen then?'*

I was so distracted I could hardly pay the girl. The shock ran all around my body, my guts were twisted with fear and for the rest of the day I barely spoke. Alissa noticed and commented that I was quiet. I just said I had work on my mind and tried to distract her attention towards something else. Throughout that day I noticed my mind lapsing, and when it did I felt completely freaked out. The thought seemed to be that if I didn't think about strangling someone that would be the moment I'd go and do it. It was similar to the twisted logic that if you don't think about breathing, you'll suddenly stop breathing and die. As weird as that.

Somehow I got through the day. The kids went to bed and I paced around the villa for an hour or so, brooding on the events tripping through my mind, until I finally lay down on the bed and tried to get some rest.

It was impossible. Mentally, I'd never felt so unwell in all my life. I thought I'd cured it, run away from it, distracted it. But it had got me good and proper.

'I'm done for,' I thought. *'I've got everything I could ever want in life and now I've got this thought and it will never, ever leave me alone again.'*

I don't know how I managed to finally fall asleep. Perhaps it was pure mental exhaustion. I woke the following morning and stumbled into the kitchen. That day I was due to fly back to the UK on business but the thought of going anywhere near the airport filled me with dread. Alissa was there, making the kids breakfast. As soon as I saw her, I burst into tears.

'Oh my God, Alissa, it's got me again,' I sobbed. 'I feel so poorly. I have to go back and I can't face it.'

She was shocked. It had been many years since I'd been like this. She tried talking to me, calming me down, reminding me that it was 'just fear'. Nothing worked.

'Look, Adam,' she said finally, 'I just don't know what to do. There's no therapist in Lanzarote. I'm sorry, baby, but you'll have to get on that plane and track down Michael when you get home.'

Michael was the first therapist I'd seen in Sheffield all those years back. It wouldn't be hard to find him, but would he even remember me and my difficulties? The only option was to give him a ring as soon as I arrived home and make an appointment to see him.

When I did finally walk through his treatment room door, he must have wondered who I was. Last time he'd seen me I was a skinny kid working at a solicitors'. Now I was an 18-stone mess, albeit a financially successful mess. I had some explaining to do, so I filled him in on the past eight years. I tried to do it without getting emotional and told him that nothing was working for me any more.

'People with OCD have these blips, Adam,' he said. 'You will recover.'

Again, he told me that it was 'just fear'.

'But it's not working,' I said. 'Telling myself that, over and over again, has lost its power. What do I do?'

Michael told me that I would be OK, that it would calm down, that I WOULD see it as just fear, given time. I felt I didn't have that time. The fear and anxiety were overwhelming me, drowning me in their own strange thoughts, rituals and compulsions. If I didn't sort this out now, I couldn't be responsible for what happened to me.

What I wasn't seeing – and perhaps what wasn't being explained to me – was that I was looking for a magic pill, a word or a sentence that would simply switch off the thoughts in my head and return me to normal. I wasn't turning to face my fear and confronting it head-on. Perhaps Michael didn't realise how much I had relied on the 'just fear' compulsion to get me through, and how devastated I was now it had lost its magic.

I left the appointment thinking *'What now?'* I had nowhere to turn, and no one to turn to. And so, over the next few hours, the anxiety and panic attacks reared up like a raging monster inside me, until the point came when I felt I had no choice but to rush myself to the local hospital as an emergency case as I was being overwhelmed with panic attack after panic attack, which give me a distressing sense that I was losing control and losing my mind.

You've read about the rest of that week, what happened to me and how close I was to ending my life, in Chapter 1. Suffice to say, it was the lowest point of my entire life. In the aftermath of that episode I couldn't work and could barely get myself out of bed. Every day felt the same – like a thick blanket of cold, wet, grey fog had enveloped me, leaving me unable to find a way out. I couldn't interact with the children, having no energy to meet their demands. That feeling fuelled the depression even further. I remember my young son knocking on my bedroom door one day, asking me to come out and play. I lay there silently, hoping he'd assume I was asleep and eventually go away. Alissa was torn between supporting me and trying to make life as normal as possible for the kids. We told them I was having headaches, and that I needed space to get better. I was still having suicidal thoughts, and feeling guilty that if I acted on these I would be leaving behind my lovely wife and children. I felt I'd be trapped in a world of despair forever. Even thinking about this now makes my stomach churn with fear. It was an awful, awful time for everyone concerned.

And yet, as I said all those pages ago and I repeat now, there was a part of me that had a glimmer of hope that I would pull through, by way of that image of my wife and children which came to my mind. And if I did survive and recover, I would help others in the same situation.

That hope was realised after I met Lauren for the first time. I so desperately wanted something to work, something that would take away all my pain and suffering forever and allow me to live a normal life. Lauren didn't usually travel to see patients but I was in no state to go to London, so she got on the train to Sheffield and met me.

'Wow, she seems young,' I thought when we shook hands. *'Will she know what she's talking about?'*

Of course she did. I couldn't have picked anyone better or more highly qualified. And she had empathy and a sense of humour too. When she left me after that first appointment, I had the feeling that this time, there might just be a solution to my problems somewhere out there ...

 Lauren: When I first met him, Adam was in an obvious state of distress because of what he was experiencing. It was clear that he was incredibly depressed, fearful and terrified that he was going mad. Not surprisingly, this can be a common presentation when I meet clients with OCD for the first time. They've been holding it together for so long that even reaching out for help is a very scary experience. Adam was very doubtful that anyone could help him and again, that's a very common perception among OCD sufferers.

As a therapist, you have to reassure clients that they will get better. This sounds an easy thing to say, and as we've seen, 'reassurance' is a tricky word when it comes to OCD and anxiety because it can be a part of the problem. However, in the context of therapy sessions it is important that the therapist offers some reassurance, because if you're experiencing OCD, particularly if it's severe, it's very normal to believe that you're beyond help. I'd go as far as to say that I've yet to meet a client with OCD who doesn't have such doubts. And yes, I've seen so many people with OCD and other anxiety problems, and they absolutely do get better. It's important to address and normalise those doubts, and for the sufferer to know that help can be sought, either in the form of a book and an approach such as the PTT approach or with a clinician or therapist who understands OCD and how to treat it.

In Chapter 5 we touched on the issue of depression that Adam had to contend with, and I mentioned that his depression was as a result of his OCD, not the other way round. Clinical depression is very common in OCD as it can exist alongside the disorder. In fact, depression is very common amongst all anxiety sufferers regardless of their diagnosis. That's perfectly understandable, because if you feel your life is falling apart and you're going crazy, and that bad things are going to happen to you, you start avoiding people, places and situations and spend all your time doing rituals and other safety behaviours. So life no longer is a pleasure, and instead is a constant source of worry, fear and dread. You feel you're not so much living your life as surviving it, and the cracks for depression to creep in as a result are wide.

Below is a checklist of signs that may indicate you are depressed:

DEPRESSION SYMPTOMS

- feeling low or sad
- loss of interest or pleasure in things
- feeling hopeless and helpless
- feeling bad about yourself
- increased tearfulness
- feeling guilty
- increased feelings of irritability
- finding it difficult to make decisions
- reduced motivation to do anything
- not getting any enjoyment out of things you used to
- having suicidal thoughts or thoughts of harming yourself
- avoiding things that you used to enjoy
- avoiding people
- increased feelings of anger or outbursts
- moving or speaking more slowly than usual

- increase or decrease in appetite or weight
- unexplained aches and pains
- disturbed sleep (for example, finding it hard to fall asleep at night or waking up very early in the morning) or sleeping more than you need (adults need on average between six and eight hours a night).[7]

If you've ticked yes to more than five of these symptoms, and you've felt like this for the past two weeks, then it is likely that you are also suffering from depression.

As I've said previously, if you have a history of clinical depression before you developed OCD or an anxiety problem, or it is so severe it is going to prevent you from getting better, you may need to have treatment for the depression first – perhaps a combination of therapy and antidepressant drugs – so that you're in a better place to tackle your OCD or anxiety. Conversely, if the OCD or anxiety problems came first and the depression has come out of the effects of OCD or anxiety problems – as we've seen with Adam – then of course it makes sense to tackle the OCD and anxiety first, in the belief that the strategies used to control OCD and anxiety will reduce the feelings of depression considerably, and probably eliminate them altogether. If you've completed the checklist above you'll have a better idea of whether you are suffering from depression. If you feel it is severe, as in you've felt like this for a long time and it is difficult to get up and do anything, or you feel suicidal, you need to seek help or advice at the time you also seek help for OCD and anxiety. In our PTT approach in Part II of this book we will look at the issue of depression in more detail.

Also in this chapter, and at the beginning of the book, we find Adam standing on a railway bridge, contemplating suicide. This is evidently a serious situation, as he felt so desperate. His suicidal thoughts were a way of trying to find a path out of his situation; if someone had offered him a pill that worked he would much rather have taken this and lived.

Remember – just because you think it doesn't mean you will do it!

7 American Psychiatric Association. (2013). *Diagnostic and Statistical Manual of Mental Disorders* (5th ed.). Arlington, VA: American Psychiatric Publishing.

Adam's response simply highlights how desperate he was to rid himself of OCD. Thoughts around suicide, especially ones that are new, are very scary and they can mix themselves in with OCD to form their own obsessions and compulsions. For example, you might have the thought of killing yourself, and attach the catastrophic meaning that you're a danger to yourself (and possibly others). So you'll avoid bridges, railway platforms, knives, tablets – anything you might associate with suicide. It's a fact that OCD mutates – it starts with an obsession over one thing and jumps around into all sorts of areas, becoming ever more complex and scary. You might begin by thinking you will harm others and jump to thoughts of harming yourself.

OCD is a bit like being in the middle of a circular room with ten doors. An intruder – your OCD – tries to get in one door and you manage to shut it. Then OCD tries another door, and another, and before long you're running round the room, desperately trying to keep all the doors shut. And of course, you just can't do that – a bit like the 'Bat the Rat' game you see at fun fairs. You belt the toy rat on his head with a mallet and within a second he's popped up somewhere else. OCD works in this 'firefighting' way, and unless you have proper treatment or follow the advice in books and programmes like this one, it will pop up again in a different form.

Just a final word about suicide. If you feel serious about killing yourself and that thought doesn't scare you, or you've made a firm plan, or you've carried out a suicide attempt before, these are clear signs that you must seek professional help as soon as possible. Don't sit hoping the thought will go away; if you feel you're in real danger you must ask for help. You can also visit www.shawmindfoundation.org for further help and information.

CHAPTER 8

THE END OF THE BEGINNING

Adam: In those first few weeks, I spoke to Lauren most days via Skype and she travelled from London twice a week. At first I wanted her to say something to me that would make me feel better immediately, i.e. something akin to, 'It's just fear, Adam.' I craved that validation of my feelings, desperately needing a new mantra to take away the pain.

With Lauren, it would never be as easy as that. After a thorough assessment, she began the recovery approach which would change my life and teach me that accepting and embracing my situation – not running away from it, creating a ritual around it or channelling it into something else – was the key to my salvation. Slowly, and over a period of months, Lauren showed me that facing my fears head-on, with no compromises, was the way forward, the only true way to a life of recovery and beyond.

At first, I didn't believe her. Who was this young academic with a New Zealand accent, and what could she possibly know about my life? The answer is: quite a lot. When I explained to her what I thought were the most shocking details of my life story, she didn't flinch. She was kind, supportive and empathetic, but also challenging. Neither was she reassuring – though of course she did assure me that I would get better. Lauren made me understand that reassurance is anxiety's ally, initially and cleverly disguising itself as your friend. Reassurance in anxiety sufferers is an addictive drug; it feels good at first, but you end up wanting a bit more each day until you get to a point where it takes over your life. You can eventually be consumed with finding reassurance and therefore battling with your thoughts and rituals every day. Lauren made me see reassurance for what it is ... a very disloyal friend and one which will ultimately betray you.

In short, she wasn't going to tell me what I wanted to hear and there were times, in the early stages, that I'd finish a conversation with her and think:

'I'm going to quit. She's not making me feel good. None of this feels right.'

Now I know that what she was doing was introducing me to the **Accept**, **Embrace**, **Control** method (detailed in our recovery approach in Part II of this book) that involved me standing up to my fears and, indeed, allowing them to come so close to me that one of us would turn tail and walk away – and it wouldn't be me.

Another block in the early stages of our therapeutic relationship was around me trying to figure out why I was still feeling so bad. I'd see her, or speak to her, and then have a couple of good days following on, and then start to feel bad again. I'd ask myself why this was happening, and it would go round and round in my head. Part of the illness around OCD and anxiety is worrying that the sensations and anxiety will never go away, even when you now understand the science behind it. This is in fact what had led me to a breakdown previously.

'What is she doing?' I'd think. *'Is she the right person? Does she understand what I've been through?'*

And so on. Until one day, when we were talking, I happened to mention that I couldn't figure out why I wasn't feeling better.

'Ironically, it's because you're trying to figure it out, Adam,' she said. 'Don't you see? OCD and anxiety thrives on you trying to understand all this. Your efforts to try and solve this and understand it completely has become another ritual. So don't. You don't need to understand it in minute detail in order to get better.'

It was another of those 'lightbulb' moments. By trying to understand it 100 per cent I was simply feeding it, in the same way I had done when I'd been running away from it. All I needed to do was accept it. It was – and is – as simple as that. It took a little while before I could truly allow myself to feel like crap but I began to recognise that I needed the bad days as much as the good ones. Feeling uncomfortable and sitting with that feeling – not fighting it – meant I was beginning to embrace my fears, and slowly but surely, I felt that the OCD and anxiety had shrunk just that little bit more each day.

The moment you accept and embrace painful thoughts, you change the game. Now you're beginning to take control, not your illness. Although I'd had doubts at the beginning, I developed faith in Lauren and – just as importantly – in myself. I knew that if I didn't run away, but instead faced my fears and accepted them, I would become desensitised to them and I would get better. Of course, there were days when I thought this approach wasn't working and I felt as though I was being tortured, but the more I sat with it, the more I faced it down. There is a saying, 'It too shall pass,' which means that just as you accept the good times will pass because you are welcoming them in, the bad times, thoughts and emotions will also pass if you accept them and let them in. All emotions and thoughts, whether good or bad, pleasant or unpleasant, are conjured up from the same part of the brain; therefore, if you accept them in, they will pass and you will become familiar with them. Just as an uplifting and very pleasant thought or emotion will dissipate over time due to you welcoming it in and embracing it, the same can be said of an unpleasant thought or emotion if you welcome it in too and don't run away from it; it too shall pass.

Eventually, I was ready to try some of Lauren's Embrace exercises. These are aimed at confronting your fears – physically, if needs be – to really bring them close and show them up for what they are. During my recovery I had a phase of becoming fixated on blinking and swallowing, worrying that I would never be able to stop thinking about doing both sensory actions once I'd started. I'd read an article on the internet about a boy whose life had been ruined by such compulsions and of course that got me thinking, 'Could it happen to me? Could it take over my life too where I wouldn't be able to stop thinking about these sensory actions which us humans have?' Far from telling me not to think about both, Lauren actively encouraged me to blink and swallow and think about these sensory actions as much and as hard as I could, again and again. Strangely enough, nothing happened; the fear and anxiety had no substance once I faced it and welcomed it in. During this stage of my recovery, she would even text me late at night to ask if I'd 'started thinking about blinking yet?'

In the past, that would have been enough to have me pacing around the house all night, but now I just laughed. And I didn't become obsessed any further about blinking or swallowing. It had actually become a joke between me and Lauren.

I also remember going to the local supermarket on my own to do some shopping. Both Lauren and Alissa thought it would be a good idea for me to just try it. It sounds like nothing, but to me it was a very big deal. Feeling that I might be on the verge of a panic attack, but also accepting that feeling and allowing it to wash over me, I managed to push a shopping trolley round the aisles and get all the groceries we needed. When I left the store I could've punched the air in triumph.

'I've done it!' I thought. 'I've really done it! And nothing bad happened to me!' For the rest of the day I couldn't stop smiling.

A big test came when we dealt with my fears of stabbing someone. Lauren had explained that I was simply reacting to a thought, nothing more, and that I'd attached a meaning to that thought, but of course this was all very well in theory. One day, in my house she went into the kitchen and brought back a knife. She handed it to me, looked me right in the eye and said:

'I want you to put this knife to my neck.'

I felt my stomach churn with nausea. Here, in one gesture, were all my fears, horrors and obsessions rolled into one. Finally, I was being given permission to do what I'd always feared I'd do, and stab someone. I'd engaged with Lauren's treatment approach fully, and I knew there would be scary situations along the path, but this was something else.

Gingerly, with trembling hands, I reached forward and put the knife to her neck. I couldn't believe this was happening. She smiled at me.

'Go on, then,' she said, 'Stab me.'

I recoiled in horror. 'I can't do that!' I screamed. 'I don't want to do it!'

After what seemed like a very long time, but was probably just five minutes, she said, 'Of course you don't, Adam. You never have wanted to do it. You were just reacting to a thought, that's all. Now you've faced that thought and you've seen it for what it is. Nothing.'

Yes, I'd faced the fear and I hadn't wanted to do it. All I needed to be was courageous, and bring it on. There were other times when Lauren encouraged me to bring on a panic attack. Try as I might, I just couldn't. But it was the element of trying to do it, of being brave and facing it, which sent it scuttling for cover.

I'm not saying any of this happened overnight. Don't get me wrong, it took weeks and months to get to the point where I could face my fears in such a way. If you're reading this and thinking, 'There's no way I could look at a spider/get my hands dirty/eat something from the floor/curse and swear out loud,' then fine. Everyone goes at their own pace, and everyone's fears and phobias are different.

But I guarantee you this: if you have been following my story, read Lauren's advice and signed up to the idea of **Accept**, **Embrace**, **Control** then you will, at some stage, face your fears head-on and by doing so, you will recover. You take control by not having control; what I mean by that is when you recognise you have a problem with OCD and anxiety, you instinctively want to find out what it is, what has caused it and how you can go about curing it. This is the wrong approach. I cannot state that loudly enough. Stop asking 'Why?' and just accept what is. No matter how you feel, accept it. It won't cure you but in my opinion it is the fundamental foundation for beginning your recovery.

 Lauren: As I've said before, anyone coming to a therapist for help around OCD and anxiety has taken a bold step. You're about to tell me things that are difficult for you to disclose, things you feel are silly, stupid, inappropriate, shocking or horrific. You're worried that I will think you're crazy. You're embarrassed and ashamed of the thoughts in your head, and the things you've done to avoid or deal with those thoughts.

It's the same with this book. You've read this far and no doubt you've come across parts of Adam's story that have made you think, 'that sounds like me'. Hopefully you've grasped the basic components of OCD and anxiety, and seen how these work with each other to create the condition. You've seen how Adam struggled with OCD and how desperate he was to find a 'solution', not realising for a long time that the solution lay within himself. He just needed the correct tools to begin his recovery.

We're now at the end of Adam's journey in this section of the book. From this point on, we will take you through your own recovery journey, building on what we've talked about so far in relation to Adam's experiences and using some modest checklists and questionnaires to help you see what's going on for you. In essence, we're giving you exactly the same therapy through our PTT approach as I would the clients who come to see me in my clinic. I'm not sitting opposite you, but in every other aspect I'm there alongside you.

Our PTT approach is based on a **Cognitive Behavioural Therapy and Compassion-Focused Approach**,[8] which is a well-established and highly effective approach to disorders such as OCD, anxiety, depression and panic attacks. At its heart it is a way of looking at the relationship between the events in our lives, how we interpret them, and our emotional and behavioural responses to them. We're looking at what links these elements together.

Cognition refers to the way we think, what we believe, how we interpret. The way we feel is our emotional response to this and the behavioural aspect is what we do about it, physically or mentally.

Take the following example: Two people are walking down the road, side-by-side. Another person approaches them and as he walks past, he laughs loudly. Now, you might be the person who thinks, 'Wonder what that was about? Who cares, it's not going to spoil my day ...'

So, the interpretation is that it's just some random event, while the associated emotional response is one of apathy. The behavioural response is to dismiss it and keep walking.

However, the other person in the pair may think this: 'What was that about? Do I look stupid? Have I got terrible hair/awful clothes/egg on my face? I need to check a mirror right away to see if everything's OK with me.' They in turn feel anxious and want to check their reflection straight away.

8 For further reading on Compassionate focused therapy please refer to; Gilbert, Paul (2010). *The Compassionate Mind: A New Approach to Life's Challenges*. Oakland, CA: New Harbinger Publications; and the Compassionate Mind Foundation homepage: www.compassionatemind.co.uk.

So you see, the other person has interpreted, emotionally responded to and acted upon the event in a completely different way. It might have completely ruined their day, whereas the first person has forgotten it in under a minute.

So it's not the event which counts, but our interpretation and response to it.

Let's have another example. I'm called in to see my boss at work. Immediately I think, 'Oh hell, I've done something wrong, I'm going to get fired. Then I'll lose my house, my friends will judge me and I'll be unemployed forever.' Consequently, I feel really down, and I find an excuse to leave work and avoid the meeting.

You, on the other hand might think: 'I've been called in to see the boss. Wow, I wonder if he/she's going to offer me a pay rise? I'm sure I'm due one. Great, I'll be able to buy those chairs I've had my eye on in the mall.' You feel excited and happy, and are planning to give yourself a reward if the pay rise happens.

We are both in the same situation, but our responses are totally different. We don't know the outcome, of course, but even if it's not one we expect we are still responsible for how we interpret it. We can't change our emotions, of course, but we can see how our interpretations affect our emotions, and how we might change our interpretation to create a more positive emotion. As we know, with OCD it's the **intrusive thought and the catastrophic meaning we give the thought**. Some people will interpret it as an odd thought, nothing more. Others will give it a meaning, and allow it to take control.

It's when our thoughts are becoming unhelpful and we feel emotionally distressed that intervention is needed.

All that said, even if you understand what's going on cognitively and rationally it doesn't mean to say that you still won't feel terrible when your OCD challenges this. If, for example, you have OCD around paedophilia, which is reasonably common (i.e. you think you're a potential child abuser and therefore a danger to children), you might understand and accept that it's only an intrusive thought you're having, but nonetheless you will still feel highly uncomfortable and anxious if you're in a swimming pool packed with kids.

But here's the thing – the more you face the fear, and go right to the heart of what is troubling you, the less you will feel anxious. It's called **'exposure'** and it's the way I work with everyone who comes to see me with anxiety. My job is to **'habituate'** you to what makes you feel most anxious. If you have anxiety around the thought that you might jump off a bridge, I will take you to that bridge. Your anxiety will be very high, but after ten minutes or so we will walk away and the anxiety will subside. The next time we do it your anxiety will still be there, but not as high as it was. The next time again, a little bit less. And so on, until you can happily walk across that bridge without the thought you'll jump off it (or if you have that thought, you're able to dismiss it as just that).

So in Part II, where you will find our PTT recovery approach, I will teach you to challenge the meaning, which then allows you to do the exposure and test it out. You can only carry out the exposure after you've challenged the cognition/catastrophic meaning, or you might just reinforce the unhelpful meaning.

In short, dealing with OCD and anxiety is not about avoiding anxiety. Quite the opposite. It's about sitting with it, embracing it, exposing yourself to it. 'Bringing it on', as Adam would say! I want to show you that a feeling, no matter how uncomfortable, will reduce the more you expose yourself to it. We **ACCEPT** the difficult thought for what it is, we **EMBRACE** it by exposing ourselves to it and sitting with it and we **CONTROL** it by becoming used to its presence and not acting on it.

It is also very important that you are **compassionate** to yourself throughout your treatment. Compassion can be defined as **'a sensitivity to suffering in yourself, and other people, and a commitment to try and alleviate and prevent it'**.[9] What this means in our approach is to recognise when you are lacking compassion to yourself, such as being self critical or feeling ashamed, and take steps to change these unhelpful responses. People with OCD and anxiety usually give themselves a very hard time, and are often very self-critical. This is not only quite punishing, but can stop people actually making progress in treatment. If every time you have a 'blip'

9 Gilbert, Paul (2010). *The Compassionate Mind: A New Approach to Life's Challenges,* Oakland, CA: New Harbinger Publications.

in your treatment, in that the thoughts might bother you more or you slip up and do a compulsion or a safety behaviour, you tell yourself you haven't tried hard enough, or that you are a failure, what effect would this have on your motivation? It is likely to make it harder to continue and you'll feel more depressed. Remember it is **not your fault** that you have OCD or anxiety. And **being kind to yourself**, rewarding yourself for successes and giving yourself a break from that self-criticism and blame will help you get better quicker. You deserve to get better, and you will get better; the ups and downs are normal and not a sign of you doing anything wrong.

There will be times in our recovery approach in Part II of this book that you will feel uncomfortable. If you didn't, the self-help measures simply wouldn't be working. Feeling uncomfortable and becoming exposed to your fear is at the core of your recovery. At first, you don't have to go all out to make yourself feel as terrible as possible – there are stages of exposure – but eventually you will need to confront that Big Thing which is bothering you. With Adam, it was the thought of killing someone, which is why I asked him to put his hands round my throat and a knife to my neck. For years, he'd had the thought that he might do this. Now he had the opportunity, he simply withdrew his hands. When he finally faced the thought that had plagued him so hard, he saw it for what it was – **just a thought, nothing more. A false fear with no substance behind it**.

Yes, this might sound scary and even turning the next page could fill you full of anxiety. But please, make that step – **pull the trigger on your OCD, anxiety, panic attacks and related depression and see what happens**. It's not easy and there may be times when you think it's too much to handle. If that's the case, take a deep breath, tell yourself that you can go forward and keep on going with the PTT approach. As I've said, you can always ask for help or support from family and friends, and within this next part of the book there is an additional section which gives a perspective on anxiety-based mental health issues from a family member's point of view.

Above all, have faith that you too can use these tools and get better.

PART II

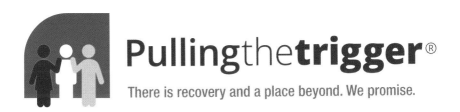

The Definitive Survival and Recovery Approach for OCD, Anxiety, Panic Attacks and Related Depression

I suffered from severe mental health issues for more than thirty years. When I brought Lauren into my life, it took just a matter of weeks to develop the building blocks for a secure and stable recovery.

Embrace this approach, embrace this journey. Your recovery is about to begin.

Adam Shaw

SECTION 1

ACCEPT

Part A: Lauren: Firstly, it's important to have an understanding of the scientific foundations provided by me in the PTT approach as this will set out the framework that will allow you to achieve your recovery. There are three main sections: **Accept**, **Embrace** and **Control**. At the end of each one of these sections is a summary where you will also find Adam's conclusion from the sufferer's point of view. This will be useful and liberating for your recovery and can be used as the benchmark for you to refer to when bringing this approach into your life.

Far from being a problem, anxiety is actually a normal human reaction to something we perceive as a threat. For example, if we're out walking and we see a big dog running towards us and barking, we are likely to react both emotionally and physiologically. Our emotional reaction might be one of worry, or even panic. Physiologically, we might start to sweat and shake, and have the feeling of our stomach turning over. No matter that the dog might just run past and pay us no attention; we have responded instinctively to what we perceive as a threat.

What do we do next? In response to the perception of threat there tends only to be three choices: fight, flight or freeze. Do we wait until the dog reaches us and fend it off, or do we run? 'Fight, flight or freeze' is an evolutionary response from prehistoric times that has (very usefully) stayed with us and is an innate, protective response which keeps us safe.

Of course, fight, flight or freeze makes more sense when the threat is obvious. A big dog running towards us has potential for threat. Even higher is the prehistoric sabre-toothed tiger prowling around outside a cave – so the cavemen inside either hide and stay very still, run away, or agree to join together and fight it off.

However, as we have developed as humans and become more sophisticated and complex in the way we live, it is often harder now to identify what a 'threat' really is. Today, threats are not just physical; they can be mental and emotional too. So while our threat system still operates as it did with our ancestors, it can be much more tricky to pin down the actual threat.

For example, the threat of losing your job could be causing you as much anxiety, relatively speaking, as the sabre-toothed tiger did to our cavemen ancestors. Although this threat doesn't mean you will die, there is the threat of losing income which might result in debt, financial hardship for your family, loss of status, the struggle to find a new job, etc. And all that is, of course, a threat to your survival in today's world. No wonder the word 'restructure' causes such a shiver down the spines of people who are told it might be happening in their workplace.

So anxiety is normal and everyone experiences it, even the most outwardly calm among us. However, it can become misplaced or misdirected, and can become a problem for us if we are experiencing it too frequently and/or too intensely in specific situations, and our appraisal system isn't managing it as well as it should.

And this is almost always down to how we interpret the threat.

Whilst this book talks about anxiety problems and OCD, and refers to anxiety as the main emotional response to these problems, there are other emotional responses that people may experience in OCD, and one in particular is **disgust**. Disgust is usually felt in forms of OCD where people are worried about being contaminated in some way or contaminating others, and it is a very strong and visceral response. Disgust is a very basic and protective response all humans have. At its core it is about keeping us safe from ingesting dangerous substances such as poison. However, just like how anxiety has evolved and now can be set off by urban threats, the disgust response can also be set off by other pollutants in our urbanised world – not just poisons, dirt and odours. It may be triggered by thoughts of contamination, or violations of our moral code, or particular type of people. So whilst we refer to anxiety as the predominant emotional response throughout this book, if you have a type of OCD in which you feel strong disgust, the same principles that we discuss throughout this book will apply to you. You can do the same steps and if it makes more sense in the practical exercises just substitute the word 'anxiety' for 'disgust'. Although it is most likely that you will feel anxiety alongside disgust too.

It may be worth re-examining a scenario we came across in the first part of this book. You're suddenly called into your manager's office for a meeting. One person may feel upset and just pack up and go home, believing that such a meeting can only be bad news. Another employee might be excited and announce to her colleagues that she'll be buying the drinks after work that evening, because this meeting could be the promotion she's hoping for. While not knowing the outcome of the meeting, the first person has avoided the situation, feels distressed and by doing so is likely to have made the situation much worse. It is more likely now that they will get into trouble for just leaving the office and not attending a meeting with their boss, the second person, while also not knowing the outcome of the meeting, has engendered goodwill among her colleagues with her positive response – which might just save her from the dreaded restructure. So our unhelpful responses to our interpretation of the situation can make the feared outcome even more likely. This is known as a **self-fulfilling prophecy**[10] – you worry something might happen so your behaviour makes it more likely that it will happen. In a diagram, it might look something like *Figure 3* on the next page.

So we see how the interpretation – the way we think about a particular situation or event – affects the emotional, physiological and behavioural reactions, and sets up patterns of thinking that reach into many other aspects of our lives.

> When you have anxiety that is interfering significantly in your work, personal or social life, it is likely that you have an anxiety disorder.

10 Merton, R. K. (1948). The self-fulfilling prophecy. *Antioch Review*, 8, 193–210.

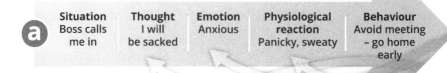

a

Situation	Thought	Emotion	Physiological reaction	Behaviour
Boss calls me in	I will be sacked	Anxious	Panicky, sweaty	Avoid meeting – go home early

b

Situation	Thought	Emotion	Physiological reaction	Behaviour
Boss calls me in	I'm getting a pay rise!	Happy, excited	Jumpy from excitement	I'll buy the drinks!

Figure 3: How we interpret events affects our emotional, physiological and behavioural responses.

So, what are the different types of anxiety problems, and how do you know which one you suffer from? It's important to say at this stage that this book does not and cannot target or treat every specific anxiety disorder there is. Some, such as Social Anxiety Disorder, need elements of specific treatment strategies that cannot be covered by the PTT approach in this particular book. For further information and help on Social Anxiety Disorder, please visit our global charity organisation at www.shawmindfoundation.org. Most anxiety problems, however, have elements in common – such as unhelpful interpretations, problematic patterns of thinking and maladaptive responses – which are included in our advice.

The following three disorders belong to the **obsessive-compulsive spectrum of disorders.**[11] That is, they have similar traits in that people experience obsessions and compulsions in each of these problems.

OBSESSIVE-COMPULSIVE DISORDER (OCD): As we have seen, OCD is a problem that can be about anything, manifesting itself in unwanted, intrusive thoughts, urges or images ('obsessions') which are recurrent and persistent, combined with repetitive behaviours

11 American Psychiatric Association. (2013). *Diagnostic and Statistical Manual of Mental Disorders* (5th ed.). Arlington, VA: American Psychiatric Publishing.

or mental acts ('compulsions') intended to deal with or avoid such obsessions. For example, intrusive thoughts about becoming contaminated with bacteria may lead to time-consuming and over-the-top hygiene practices, including excessive handwashing and showering.

HEALTH ANXIETY: In less sympathetic times this was known as 'hypochondria'. This is a form of OCD. It involves obsessions about illness or falling ill and repetitive behaviour (compulsions) seeking reassurance via frequent visits to the doctor or, increasingly now, self-diagnosis on the internet. For example, someone might worry obsessively about having a brain tumour, excessively monitor their health for signs of deterioration and make frequent trips to their doctor to ask for tests and MRI scans.

BODY DYSMORPHIC DISORDER (BDD): Here, a person worries excessively about one or more slight or perceived defects in their appearance that are not noticeable or appear very insignificant to others. They then perform repetitive behaviours and mental acts to disguise these problem areas. For example, someone worrying that their facial pores may be too big may check their appearance obsessively in the mirror, wear heavy make-up to cover them, hide behind scarves and hats, seek unnecessary cosmetic procedures and constantly compare their skin to other people's skin.

The following disorders are considered **Anxiety Disorders**[12] in which people experience excessive fear and anxiety in situations which have a low level of threat, and this results in behavioural disturbances. Although anxiety and fear play a big role in OCD, the OCD disorders also have the obsessions and compulsions which help differentiate them from these disorders.

GENERALISED ANXIETY DISORDER (GAD): People with GAD might sometimes be described as 'worriers'. A bit harsh, perhaps, but GAD is defined by excessive and uncontrollable worry for reasonably long periods of time, and people find it difficult to control the worry. The worry can jump from subject to subject and can lead to worry about worry itself. People will also have physical symptoms such as restlessness, irritability, muscle tension and sleep problems.

12 American Psychiatric Association. (2013). *Diagnostic and Statistical Manual of Mental Disorders* (5th ed.). Arlington, VA: American Psychiatric Publishing.

SOCIAL ANXIETY DISORDER (SOCIAL PHOBIA): A fear of how you will be scrutinised or judged in public. It can apply to any situation where you feel 'on show' and at risk of being negatively judged by others. Sufferers avoid interacting with other people or specific social situations, or engage in safety behaviours when they are in the feared situation. For example, someone worrying that other people might find them boring or dull might drink too much alcohol at a party to feel more relaxed and confident, and to stop themselves worrying so much (but this in fact makes them worry more the next day because they can't clearly remember what they said or how they acted).

PHOBIAS: This is an intense fear of a specific object or situation, such as snakes, spiders, flying or open spaces. The response to the object or situation is excessive and disproportionate to the actual risk, and may cause the sufferer to avoid everyday things or situations. Although some phobias may be more common, such as phobias about flying or spiders, you can in fact develop a phobia about anything.

PANIC DISORDER: People experience panic attacks, which are feelings of sheer terror that strike suddenly with no warning and reach a peak of fear within minutes. Panic attacks cause people to worry that they might lose control of themselves in some way or may be having a heart attack or mental breakdown. While panic attacks are common in all the anxiety and obsessive-compulsive disorders, in Panic Disorder the sufferer fears having more panic attacks and goes to great lengths to avoid situations in which they worry they might have a panic attack. This can even leave some people housebound as they worry that as soon as they leave their house they may have a panic attack. As we've seen in Adam's story, panic attacks are a result of heightened anxiety, and regularly occur among sufferers of any anxiety problem. It is the fear of having more panic attacks which gives the diagnosis of Panic Disorder.

While this is not an exhaustive list of anxiety problems, it covers some of the main disorders and their specific features. It's also important to say that even if you as the reader don't meet the specific criteria for an anxiety disorder or an obsessive-compulsive disorder, you may still experience anxiety which interferes with your life; thus, reading about the PTT approach will be helpful.

What causes such anxiety disorders? Well, we don't know exactly – as we have previously mentioned, it can be a combination of responses to the environment or events, changes in brain chemistry, our genes, our early experiences in life. What we can say, however, is that it is not as a result of weakness or faults of character. Sufferers with anxiety are very often hard on themselves, blaming themselves for their problems. The fact is, we all need emotional responses in our lives. Emotions are a cornerstone of human existence; they act as our guides in life and without them we are cold and robotic. As we've explained, fear and anxiety are normal responses that people need in order to keep safe. So it is normal to have strong feelings or emotions; it is how we respond and interpret these which makes the difference between 'normal' and 'problem' responses.

Depression as a stand-alone condition is not covered by the PTT approach. For more information and help on depression as a stand-alone condition, please visit www.shawmindfoundation.org. However, it is the case that depression can, and often does, arise as a result of obsessive-compulsive problems and anxiety difficulties. As we've said, that's hardly surprising. Your life has been so debilitated by OCD and anxiety that it's no surprise that you are unable to find pleasure in life and have therefore become depressed. That said, if depression was a pre-existing condition – i.e. it was there before OCD or an anxiety problem – or it is so severe it will prevent you from being able to get better, it has to be treated separately. OCD and anxiety-related depression is covered in these pages, and it's very often the case that if you're effectively managing your OCD or anxiety problem, the depression side of it lessens accordingly.

So for the purposes of the PTT approach, we are looking primarily at OCD, anxiety, panic attacks and related depression, but all of the above can be treated using Cognitive Behavioural Therapy (CBT). However, you will find some of the strategies suggested in here will help with other anxiety problems too.

Let's have a quick recap of what our **Cognitive Behavioural Therapy and Compassion-Focused Approach** is, because this forms the basis of our unique PTT approach – the combination of **Accept**, **Embrace** and **Control** – we are using to tackle your anxiety problem. At its heart, CBT is the study of the relationship between things that happen in our lives, how we interpret them and our physiological, emotional and behavioural responses to them. We're looking for what links these elements up – what we describe as 'cognition', the way we think, what we believe, how we interpret things. The 'physiological' is our bodily reaction, the 'emotional' is our feeling response to this and the 'behavioural' is what we do about it, physically or mentally. CBT is the best treatment that we have to date for anxiety and obsessional disorders; it is evidence-based and it hands over the tools of treatment, recovery and maintenance of that recovery to the individual. So the clinicians are NOT the secret holders of information! We are meant to impart it and encourage people to share it. Think of this approach as a toolbox – you may find some of the exercises and challenges to be very useful, others less so, but please read through the whole PTT approach first before deciding which is which.

Finally, let me say something about **compassion**. To overcome your anxiety and/or obsessional problem, you need to have compassion for yourself, even as you are motivated to make changes in your life. In psychology, compassion is defined as the feeling you get when you want to alleviate someone's suffering.

In this case, that someone is you.

To change, we have to take a journey that is non-judgemental and does not involve blame. We must be kind to ourselves during our journey; with anxiety and obsessional problems it is very common to be self-attacking and self-critical, and ashamed and embarrassed of having the problems we've described. These things will hold you back from getting better.

> You are a worthwhile person and deserve to be treated in a compassionate, warm and supportive way. Treating yourself in a kind and non-judgemental way is incredibly important and helpful for your recovery.

On your journey through this recovery approach there may be times when you feel that it isn't going as well as you'd hoped, or it feels too hard. But if you give yourself time, patience and compassion, this will result in the courage you need to overcome such roadblocks.

 Part B: Lauren: Now we've looked at various anxiety and obsessive disorders and have introduced the principles of CBT, which is used to treat them, let's have a look at what YOU want to get from our **PTT** treatment approach.

The answer – without wanting to put words in your mouth – is that you want a life free from the anxiety and/or obsessions that currently trouble you. Of course you do. But for this bigger thing to happen, we need to break down your goals into smaller, more easily digested pieces. This way, you will really be able to see what is going on, accepting that it is a problem for you and seeing it for what it is, which will help you move on to the next stage of recovery.

In my clinical practice, during the initial appointment with clients where I am trying to understand their anxiety or obsessional problem with them, I will always ask:

How is the problem you're suffering from interfering in your life?

Perhaps you can write your answer in the box below. Think about how it affects you in work, at home, within your relationship and social life ...

Table 1: *How my problem interferes with my life.*

> My problem interferes in my life in the following way(s) ...

Let's think back to how difficult life was for Adam during his period with OCD. At school he was unable to achieve the grades he should have done. Later, his career as a pilot was ruined and although he went on to be successful in another field, there were times he was unable to work and his family suffered as a result of his severe episodes of anxiety. The interference of OCD and anxiety in his life was very high. You may not feel that your anxiety intrudes upon your own life with such regularity or severity, but it may be that the times it feels difficult are becoming more frequent. You may have tried to accommodate it so it doesn't feel like it is a problem on a daily basis – but you will have changed plans or made compromises because of it, just like Adam.

We will look a little more closely at how your situation has become increasingly difficult. Below is a series of questions that will help to break down your difficulty into manageable parts, challenging you to think about each stage of your anxiety. The reason for doing this is to help you see the links between the situation and your thoughts, feelings, physiological reactions and behaviour, which we looked at in the previous chapter.

Table 2: *Working out my own problematic thoughts, feelings and responses.*

When did you last experience your problem? Where were you?

Describe what happened.

What was going through your head at the time? What were you thinking? What did you think was the worst thing that could possibly happen from this?

How did you feel emotionally? (Angry/sad/fearful/worried/excited/ashamed, etc.?)

How did you feel in your body? (Sweaty/blurred vision/stomach turning over/edgy/keyed up, etc.?)

How did you react – what did you do? Did you avoid anything or seek reassurance from anyone? (Remember that your reaction can also be a mental reaction occurring in your head such as a chant, saying a certain phrase or neutralising – trying to replace an unhelpful thought with a neutral or a 'good' one.)

What were the consequences of your reaction? (Even though it might reduce your anxiety immediately, what are the other consequences of your behaviour? E.g. I avoided giving a work presentation.)

Hopefully, you will now see that how you interpreted the situation (the situation being the 'trigger' point) has affected your subsequent reactions towards it. In therapy, we usually call these interpretations '**unhelpful thinking**' and when we step back from and reflect on the situation, we usually see **patterns of unhelpful thinking** emerging. Unsurprisingly, unhelpful thinking doesn't always follow the logical pattern set out above; i.e. it is not always prompted by 'something' happening which in turn prompts a sequence of events. We might just have an intrusive thought, or have a feeling of dread first, or physiological sensations such as shaking and sweating. On their own, these might not make much sense but the 'creeping' sensation of things not being right is real enough. We might know we are avoiding something at work, but don't really understand why. Yet we know there are triggers making us feel this way.

If this is the case for you, then start with understanding:

- What is the situation you are in when you start feeling uncomfortable? What is it you were thinking about when you started feeling that way?

  or

- What is it in your behaviour that is unhelpful – what are you not doing (avoiding) or doing that is causing you problems?

And you can always work backwards to see what it is you are really worried about.

Another way to figure out what is going on for you in certain situations is to look at the diagram below and see how thoughts, feelings, responses and behaviours are all connecting to produce a **'vicious cycle'** of unhelpful thoughts.[13]

Figures 4 & 5: *The interaction of our thoughts, emotions, behaviours and physiological reactions.*

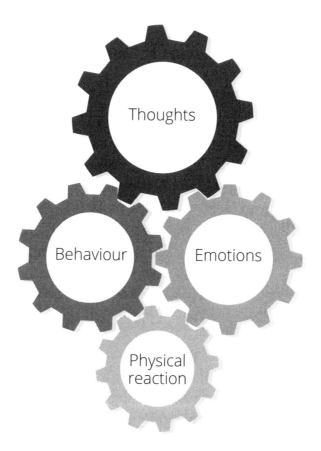

Let's model this around someone who worries about turning off electrical appliances before leaving the house and has recently read about a house fire which was caused by a faulty appliance.

13 Beck, A. T. & Emery, G., with Greenberg, R. L. (1985). *Anxiety Disorders and Phobias: A Cognitive Perspective.* New York: Basic Books.

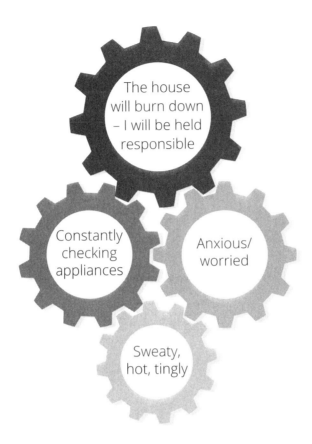

So you see how all these things are connected.

As we said before, sometimes we just get a feeling of dread and it can be difficult to know what we are actually worried about. For example, someone might have intrusive thoughts about being a paedophile, but what they are actually worried about is that other people will think they are a paedophile or weird for having these intrusive thoughts, not that they are actually a paedophile. Someone might have thoughts about harming their newborn baby, but what they are really worried about is that they are not a fit parent for having these thoughts. Someone might have intrusive thoughts about upsetting their boss or doing the wrong thing at work, but what they are really worried about is being thought of as stupid by other people. Someone might have intrusive thoughts about coming into contact with blood; it is not infectious diseases they are worried about, but that they won't ever get rid of these thoughts and that they will be driven mad by them. It is not always obvious what the core worry is – but you will know it when you get there as it will fit and make sense to you. To assist, have a look at the box below and fill in the answer:

> **Our worries take many forms. What do you think are your core worries? Write them down below:**

Table 3: My core worries.

One way to try to understand what it is that you are actually thinking at the time is by using a technique I describe as 'why not?', which requires that you question yourself at each stage of the process until you get to the true reason for the anxiety. To illustrate this, let's look at the example of a person who doesn't want to make a presentation at work, see Figure 6 opposlte.

Eventually, by asking yourself 'why not?' the core thinking at the centre of the anxiety is revealed. In this case, the employee worries that other people think they are stupid and they are not fit to be in their present job. This thought may or may not be true, but it feels very real. When you next have an anxious feeling or an intrusive thought, work through this series of questions to see what lies at the bottom. You might be surprised to learn what it actually is that you are worried about! Try doing it in more than one situation to see if it is the same thing you are worried about in all situations, or whether you have other core worries too.

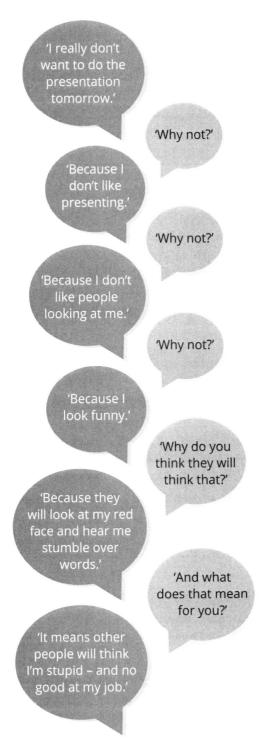

Figure 6: *Example of 'Why Not?' questioning.*

Now you have some idea of how anxiety is interfering, let's conclude this section by seeing if we can set some goals for **accepting** and managing it. Adam's short-term goal was to get through each day without worrying whether he would harm someone. In the medium term he wanted to gain an understanding of his anxiety problem and feel comfortable and successful at work without anxiety eating him up. His goal for the long term was to live a happy, stable life in the company of his family – and to inspire others to feel the same way, free of OCD and anxiety.

What are your short-, medium- and long-term goals? Perhaps you'd like to get out of the house you feel you're trapped in and take a short walk, or drive to the swimming pool to go for a swim? You might want to go to work without feeling the need to drive home and check you've turned the cooker off. Maybe you'd like to repair the relationship that has been damaged by your anxiety, or change jobs? In the long term, perhaps your aim is very similar to Adam's: using the techniques you've picked up from us to manage your anxiety better and live a happier, healthy life.

To identify your goals, please fill in the box on page 115. To help you, think about achieving the short-term goals when you've read this book, the medium-term ones within six months and the long-term ones at any distant point in the future you feel comfortable with.

MY GOALS ARE ...

Short-term:

Medium-term:

Long-term:

Table 4: My goals for treatment.

Part C: Lauren: As we know, not all thoughts are created equally. What I might think about something is highly likely to be different from the way you think about it. I might forget to call my mother and think, 'Oh well, not to worry, she'll be around tomorrow.' You might think, 'I'm such a bad son/daughter for forgetting. It just proves what a terrible person I am.'

We have different types of thoughts. We've already discussed intrusive thoughts, which are uncontrollable thoughts that can occur frequently and can cause us distress, but remember – everyone has these! These intrusive thoughts fit into a category known as 'automatic thoughts' – thoughts that pop into our head, such as when looking in the fridge you might think 'I need to remember to buy some milk.' These are usually non-threatening and occur a lot during the day. In fact, as we have mentioned, it is estimated that we have around 50,000 to 70,000 thoughts a day. Personally, I can only usually remember around a dozen of mine by bedtime. So what makes us remember any particular intrusive or automatic thought? That would be our interpretation of that thought and the emotional and behavioural response we have to it.

There are other types of thoughts we have but probably are less aware of as they aren't always present in our daily routines or in the front of our minds. These are called **rules or assumptions**, and **core beliefs**.[14] These can often set us up for having troubling intrusive or automatic thoughts. Rules and assumptions are contingency-based rules we live by. For example, we might think *'it is important to be liked by others, otherwise it will mean that I am failing in some way'*. This might lead us to having daily intrusive or automatic thoughts in which we worry about offending people. Another example might be *'it is important to be careful with your belongings, otherwise it means you are ungrateful and careless'*, and therefore someone might have daily worries about losing items. These rules help us make sense of the world, our place in it and how we should go about behaving. They can be both helpful and unhelpful. For example, I might have a rule that *'it's OK for people to dislike me as long as I am being true to myself and my own views'* and thus will be less likely to be paralysed by the fear of offending people.

14 Beck, J. S. (2011). *Cognitive Behavior Therapy: Basics and Beyond* (2nd ed). New York: Guilford.

We also all hold strong, often rigid beliefs about ourselves, other people and the world around us – core beliefs – that we hang onto throughout our lives. We might see the world as a generally dangerous, unwelcoming place and never want to venture much beyond our street or our town. On the other hand, we might see it as a place of wonder, there to be explored despite the potential for danger. We might think other people are careless and incompetent, and that only we can do things properly. Or perhaps we're happy to allow other people to take responsibility for things, believing they know more than us.

Of course, we all hold these beliefs with different levels of conviction or strength. And as we've seen, it's not just the thoughts we have on a daily basis, but the **interpretation** of them which often comes from these core beliefs or assumptions. If you believe the world is a dangerous place and you're happy to stay in your neighbourhood and never fly anywhere else, then fine. If, however, you long to visit a friend or relative in another country and you can't because of a belief that something will happen to you, **then your thinking is unhelpful, whether it is an automatic thought, intrusive thought, rule or assumption or core belief**. If your worries and anxieties are strong and regular, and you feel panicky or uncomfortable every time you think about or experience the trigger which sets them off, these are indications that something is wrong.

So we can use our feelings as a guide to check for a problem in the way we think. If you feel very anxious, depressed, frustrated, angry etc. then it might be worth going back to examine the thoughts that you had at the time. Sometimes these problems are called '**thinking errors**' as errors are considered 'wrong', whereas everybody has patterns of these thinking problems, and it wouldn't make sense if we were all wrong in the way we were thinking! Therefore, I would prefer to use the term '**thinking problems**'. In therapy, we come across many of these thinking problems. On the next page are a few of the more common ones:

CATASTROPHISING

Thinking the worst-case scenario about every event, no matter how minor. *'If I leave the house without checking the window, someone will definitely break into the house.'*

THOUGHT-ACTION FUSION[15]

Having such a thought means it is more likely to happen, or it means that thinking about the action is as bad as actually doing it. **'***Because I had this thought it means that I am more likely to hurt someone, or that I must really want to hurt someone.'*

MAGNIFIED DUTY

Believing you are 100 per cent responsible or have an increased responsibility for things, discounting the fact that other people may share responsibility.[16] *'I am the only person responsible for making sure the window is secure, therefore if anything bad happens it will be 100 per cent my fault.'*

PERSONALISING

Thinking that everything is your fault, even when you couldn't have had anything to do with it. *'My team lost, I'm a jinx – I shouldn't have been at the match!'*

BLACK AND WHITE THINKING or ALL-OR-NOTHING THINKING

Experiences or things are only categorised as one way or another, often as good or bad, with no in-between. *'I broke my diet rule as I ate two biscuits so I have ruined the whole diet completely.'*

CRYSTAL BALL THINKING / FORECASTING THE FUTURE

Thinking you can predict the future, or living as if the future has happened. *'I know exactly what will happen if I go to this meeting ...'*

---

15 Shafran, R., Thordarson, D. S. & Rachman, S. (1996). Thought-action fusion in obsessive compulsive disorder. *Journal of Anxiety Disorders*, 10(5), 379–91.
16 Salkovskis, P. M., Wroe, A. L., Gledhill, A., Morrison, N., Forrester, E., Richards, C. & Thorpe, S. (2000). Responsibility attitudes and interpretations are characteristic of obsessive compulsive disorder. *Behaviour Research and Therapy*, 38(4), 347–72.

JUMPING TO CONCLUSIONS

Making a judgement, usually negative, even when there is little or no evidence for it. *'Someone's texting during my presentation: they must all think I'm very boring ...'*

'SHOULD BE' and 'OUGHT TO BE'

Thinking things HAVE to be a certain way, or people (including you) SHOULD behave in a particular way. *'I SHOULD get 100 per cent in every test'*; *'People OUGHT TO BE friendly all the time.'*

GUARANTEES ABOUT THE FUTURE

Needing everything to be guaranteed or the outcome of events to be known, despite this being impossible. *'I need to know 100 per cent that something bad won't happen in the future.'*

EMOTIONAL REASONING

Basing things on how you feel, rather than reality. *'I just FEEL that something bad will happen.'*

PERCEIVED CONTROL or SUPERSTITIOUS THINKING

Believing you have control over events or outcomes that you cannot actually influence. *'If I do all these chores right, then my family will be safe.'* This can sometimes be known as **MAGICAL THINKING** in its extreme form: *'If I don't touch the light switch six times then my grandmother in Australia will become ill or die.'*

OVERESTIMATION OF LIKELIHOOD OR PROBABILITY

Believing an event to be imminent and extremely likely to take place despite how unlikely it is in reality. *'If I take this plane trip, it is going to crash.'*

MIND READING

Believing that you know what other people are thinking, despite having no evidence for it. *'I know that my colleague thinks I am stupid.'*

Table 5: Common thinking problems.

This list is a careful selection of the many thinking problems people engage in, and the ones I see most in anxiety and obsessional problems. Do any of these apply to you? Are there thinking problems you have which you feel might be causing you unhelpful thoughts? If so, write them in the box below.

Remember, more than one thinking problem can apply to each problematic thought! And if you are not sure when you might be doing one of these thinking problems, use a time recently when you felt anxious, worried, or depressed, and you will probably find that you experienced at least one thinking problem.

A 'trigger' event – something happening in your external world or an intrusive thought in your head – can set off unhelpful thinking

---

My worry or problematic thoughts are:

The thinking problems that apply to these worries are:

Table 6: *Identifying my own thinking problems.*

interpretations, prompting emotional, physiological and behavioural reactions. We have seen how a vicious cycle of anxiety develops in the previous chapter. We might also call this an unhelpful cycle, and very often people become stuck, as all elements of the cycle spin and interact, reinforcing the anxiety. This vicious cycle model applies equally to OCD or other obsessive problems, anxiety problems and panic, and being caught up in this cycle can be a profoundly disturbing and distressing experience.

If you have OCD or another anxiety problem it's likely that you will **Catastrophise** or feel a sense of **Magnified Duty** and **Seek Guarantees about the Future**, or try and exert **Perceived Control**. Your emotional responses might involve anxiety, fear, worry, doubt and panic. Your behavioural responses are most likely to be **safety-seeking actions**, **avoidance** – the absence of active responses, observable compulsions and rituals – and **mental compulsions** which include **rumination** (mentally dwelling on the problem), **mental checking** for signs of danger and **mental rewinding** of events to see if you must take responsibility for them (for example, running a recent car journey back through your mind to make sure you didn't hit anyone) or to ensure that you haven't done something wrong. They may also be **ritual-based**, such as Adam's 'just fear' mantra. Behavioural responses are, of course, things we do or don't do to rid ourselves of anxiety in a bid to feel better.

As we know, such behaviours only reinforce anxiety. They can also make your physical situation worse too. For example, if your anxiety is around going to the dentist, your catastrophic interpretation of this trigger/event is that it will be painful and unpleasant, and you won't cope with the pain and anxiety of being there. However, if you have a toothache and you avoid the dentist, the physiological consequence is that it will become worse, perhaps requiring more serious treatment at a later stage. If your anxiety is around harming your children in some way, one of the consequences might be that you avoid the children and subsequently they don't get the care they need.

These are what we might call the **Unintended Consequences** of a behavioural response to an anxiety problem.

Think about the **unintended consequences** of your behavioural responses (including avoidance) and write them down here:

Table 7: *The unintended consequences of my avoidance behaviour.*

With anxiety, there is also the threat of anxiety itself. Let's say we're stuck again with the fear of the dentist. You've avoided the appointment time and time again, but the thought of going to the dentist and the emotions surrounding it are still swirling around your head. Then you begin to think, *'Oh no, I'm thinking about this again. Why do I keep thinking this way? Am I losing my mind?'* or *'I will go mad with all the worry.'* Similarly, you can have **OCD about OCD**, **panic about panic** and **depression about depression**. And so the vicious cycle keeps spinning.

It's also common for anxiety to jump from one thing to another. If you managed to successfully put one worry out of your mind, within a short space of time you're highly likely to find yourself worrying about something else. For example, you've stopped worrying about locking the front door – but now you keep worrying about whether you said something inappropriate to your boss. Adam wondered if he might worry that he would harm his firstborn child, but that worry mutated into one in which his wife and daughter would disown him if he harmed someone else and was sent to prison. The content of the worry can change, and that is normal because worry simply doesn't want to go away and will not go away without help, so it will make it hard for you.

At this stage, it is vital to know one thing: **we cannot change or control the triggers that cause our anxiety, internal or external, because they are part of everyday life**. When you try to change them, or push them away, all you are doing is reinforcing the unhelpful thinking around them, causing the vicious cycle of anxiety to spin faster and longer.

> Everyone has intrusive thoughts, or experiences life events that are beyond our control. To manage anxiety and obsessional problems, you have to ACCEPT this as fact.

From time to time we all face challenges in life, or experience strange, unpleasant and downright weird thoughts. This is all part of human existence. Understanding and **accepting** this is the case, and knowing that everyone – rich or poor – experiences challenging thoughts or life events is the key to going forward and managing your anxiety problem. As Adam states, 'Acceptance doesn't mean curling into a ball and telling yourself you're finished.' It simply means that you're **accepting your state of mind, as it is at the moment**. Accepting means not judging. To move on you need to accept, not judge yourself or the thoughts. This is much easier to do once you've understood and used the PTT approach.

If you understand that your anxiety is the result of an interpretation of a trigger, which has led to thinking problems and a vicious cycle of anxiety not rooted in reality, you can now begin to **accept** this and move to a stage where you can do something about it. I don't mean in terms of 'fight' or 'struggle'. We've seen how fighting and struggling has the opposite effect, in that it makes the anxiety cycle spin faster. On the contrary, I encourage sufferers to accept their thoughts and emotions before embracing them by going towards the cause of their anxiety rather than stepping away from it.

> By accepting and embracing our thoughts and feelings, we learn ultimately to control them by not having to control them.

Accepting our thoughts and our feelings can feel very uncomfortable and counter-intuitive to some extent. When things feel uncomfortable or distressing, our first instinct is to solve or avoid the problem, and this message is reinforced by everyday living. Think of all the advertisements you are bombarded with on a daily basis – if you have a physical pain, fix it with a pill; if you have hair loss, fix it with this treatment ... and so on. However, this does not work in anxiety, as we have seen. So it is important to know that however uncomfortable your thoughts or feelings are, they are **not permanent**. They will not last forever, and will change hour by hour, day by day, week by week. Think of how you felt when you woke up this morning. I guarantee that you will be feeling differently by this evening (it could be you feel worse or better than this morning), but the point is that it will be different from how you were feeling this morning, whether a different feeling or different intensity of the same feeling. All thoughts and all feelings are impermanent and do not last forever, and they will change over time.

In Section 2 of the PTT approach (**Embrace**) we will look at ways of challenging unhelpful thoughts and interpretations to help you see that anxiety is almost never based on reality.

SUMMARY

Lauren: In this section we'll recap everything we've learned so far about anxiety-based illnesses, then Adam will add his conclusion about **accepting** anxiety. We know there is a lot to take in, and while our **PTT** approach is essentially not a complicated one, there are building blocks to understand and accept your anxiety problem before we move on to the next, more practical stage of our treatment approach.

Remember, anxiety and fear are less of a problem and more of a human condition that applies to everyone. **Fear is the emotional reaction to real or perceived imminent danger. Anxiety is a response to what we anticipate as a threat**, and these can be very useful responses in the right situation. Remember the example we gave about the dog running towards you, and the 'fight, flight or freeze' mechanism. Panic attacks are an acute experience of fear and anxiety responses, and happen across all anxiety and obsessional disorders.

Threats are not just about large dogs. They can be about redundancy, divorce, death, loss, illness and everything else we see as a challenge to everyday existence. But threats only become a problem when we seem to be mismanaging them. This is all down to **whether we interpret the event, situation or thought as a highly likely or probable threat and seek to remove any likelihood of it happening in the future**.

For example, many people accept death as an inevitable part of life. While they'd rather it didn't happen to them, they know that one day it will. Others, however, see death as the biggest threat in life, and do everything to avoid it (and by doing so, ironically don't really live life as they should. As they say, 'If you tiptoe through life, you arrive safely at death!') This is what we mean by **interpretation** and **mismanaging our responses**.

We don't really know precisely what causes all anxiety disorders. We know there are likely genetic elements involved, brain structures and neurochemical components, early life experiences, and/or responses to environment or life changes – but we don't actually need to know the cause to solve the problem. The fact is, we have to **accept** anxiety as normal; it is our (mis)interpretation of things as threats, and our responses to anxiety which causes problems. And to get better, we must have **compassion** for ourselves. Continually blaming or being hard on ourselves is of no help at all. **Remember: this is not your fault. You do not need to blame anyone or anything for this problem.** However, **accepting** it as a problem allows you to move on and embrace the next steps to overcome it.

Next, we looked at your specific anxiety or obsessional problem and asked you:

- What triggers it?
- How do you think about it?
- How does it make you feel in your body?
- How do you feel emotionally?
- How do you react to it?

We got you to look at your trigger points – external events, feelings or unhelpful thoughts – and, by asking you how you reacted, tried to discover how you interpreted the threat. We identified these interpretations as **unhelpful thinking patterns**. By looking at these thoughts we attempted to identify the core worries – the ones which are causing all the trouble.

We also looked at your emotional, physiological and behavioural responses to these unhelpful thoughts, and showed you how they all contribute to go round and round to form a **vicious cycle of anxiety**.

We also asked you to identify your short-, medium- and long-term goals. While we're not about tick boxes and targets, having a focal point in a future free from your anxiety-based or obsessional illness is extremely useful. **You will get better, and you will live the life you want to live**.

In Part C we looked at different types of thoughts we have – those which you cling onto for dear life. Some might not trouble you, such as the political party you vote for or the religious views you hold. Others, however, might actually prevent you from living a full and happy life. Again, it is all down to **interpretation**. Examining our thinking leads us to identify **thinking problems**. We looked at some of the more common ones and saw how these thinking problems found in our thoughts or interpretations of an event triggered such a pattern, leading to anxiety and its vicious cycle.

What we do, or don't do, in reaction to our interpretations of thoughts and events, helps to spin the cycle faster, leaving us trapped in our anxiety. But of course, such triggers – intrusive thoughts or external events – are around us all the time. We cannot change this situation; all we can do is **ACCEPT** that we all experience such triggers, and go on to **EMBRACE** these by challenging both the meaning that lies behind them for us and our behavioural responses. Only this way will we learn to **CONTROL** our response to anxiety, and therefore begin to feel better about it.

In **ACCEPTING** our thoughts and feelings, however uncomfortable, we know that feelings and thoughts are **impermanent** and **do not last forever**.

ADAM'S CONCLUSION: ACCEPTANCE

 Adam: When I first met Lauren and she told me that, rather than fighting my OCD and anxiety, I'd be better off accepting it, I thought she might be joking.

'What a cop-out!' I told myself when she'd gone. 'How can I accept something I've been fighting all these years? I need to find a solution to my problem – anything else is just giving in.'

I saw my illness as a 'fight', a 'battle' and a 'struggle', and for all my life I'd responded by putting up my fists and trying to fight back. To be told to lay down my arms and accept the situation as it was seemed ridiculous. There was no way I was going to 'accept' anything about OCD and anxiety.

At that point, however, I was so poorly and so in need of help that I had to trust someone. Lauren is one of the leading therapists in anxiety and I was very fortunate to bring her into my life as my therapist, so if I couldn't trust her I couldn't trust anyone. She was my last chance. Lauren didn't promise me a miracle cure, but neither did she seem untrustworthy on first meeting her. There was a part of me that said, 'Stick with this, and see what happens ...' And I'm so glad that I did because if I'd carried on fighting, battling and struggling I might not be writing these words today. At one point during the first couple of sessions, Lauren said:

'Adam, everything you thought would be helpful over the last thirty years in trying to fight your mental health issues – has any of it ever worked?'

'I suppose so,' I replied, 'but only temporarily.'

'OK,' she said, 'then you've been trying to figure this out for more than thirty years and it's made you very ill. So why not try it another way – even if it feels uncomfortable?'

So I thought about it, and just decided to give it a go. As a fellow sufferer, you might have had the same thoughts about this book – but you've stuck with us and made it this far. Perhaps what you've read, particularly in this 'Pulling the Trigger' section, has made you feel uncomfortable but please stay with us. You too might think it strange that we're asking you to accept your illness for what it is, and I understand that. But accepting (with embracing and controlling, which we'll learn about in the next sections) in my view is the only way you will get better. Let me explain why.

Acceptance is NOT about giving in. It is about allowing your mind to be how it wants to be, to go where it wants to go, to let in what it wants to let in – thoughts both welcome and unwelcome. It's about saying, 'This is my state of mind, these are the thoughts I am having, this is how I am feeling. I'm accepting it for what it is. I might feel bad, but I accept that.' Until you start 'accepting' you are always going to carry the burden of the thoughts and feelings around with you, and over time those thoughts and feelings will get heavier and heavier, which can lead us to those dark places I have already discussed previously in my personal story.

If you hold a glass of water in your hand for a short period of time, it is of course relatively easy and painless to hold. Carry on holding that same glass of water for a sustained and longer period and with no respite, then that glass of water begins to become heavier and heavier, and the burden of carrying it becomes greater. Even though the glass of water is relatively light, you have continued to hold it for so long that it's becoming heavier and heavier and is taking its toll on your arm muscles; your physical limits have been stretched and the muscle in your arm simply gives up! The same applies to your mind with thoughts; if you continue to carry the intrusive/anxious thought by battling with it, judging it, trying to understand it, rectifying it, and developing a compulsion to try and make peace with it, then you are in effect continuously carrying it just like the glass of water. The mind will only be able to carry it for so long, as I found out when the thoughts just got too heavy and the panic attacks kicked in. Accept your thoughts and state of mind for what they are in that moment, in that hour, day or even that week. Put the glass of water down and go about your day.

Acceptance isn't about fighting, battling or anything else other than having the courage to accept what is. Fight, as we will see, is a very close **ally** of anxiety. Anxiety loves nothing more than a good battle, because that's where it **gains** its power. Acceptance is an enemy of anxiety because it **diminishes** its power. Having the courage to accept your situation is the polar opposite of battling it. Below is a table of anxiety's allies and enemies. Do keep referring to this; it's a very useful guide to what is helpful and what is not during your recovery, and I wish I'd had something like this when I was starting to get better.

 Anxiety's Allies   **Anxiety's Enemies**

Anxiety's Allies	Anxiety's Enemies
Seeking constant reassurance	Taking risks with your anxieties
Performing rituals or compulsions	Telling your anxiety to 'come on in'
Running away from your anxiety	Having courage to face your fears
Questioning your state of mind	Accepting your state of mind
Fighting or battling your thoughts	Sitting with your thoughts until they pass
Feeling uncomfortable about feeling uncomfortable	Being OK with not feeling OK
Fearing anxiety	Doing everyday things despite feeling anxious
Avoiding everyday things because you feel anxious	Being kind and forgiving to yourself
Trying to 'solve' or figure everything out	Not judging yourself for having these thoughts, feelings or behaving in this way
Worrying that you will go mad with worry	
Self-criticism and self-blame	

Table 8: Anxiety's allies and enemies.

So if you accept your state of mind and emotional state, you are owning it for what it is. You're not forcing it to do anything other than allow anxiety to come and go. And yet, even when I started to understand the concept of **'Accept'** there were times it didn't feel right. I reverted to type, put up a fight and guess what? I felt twice as bad as I did when I was just accepting my state of mind. So eventually I saw it as a shrug of the shoulders, a 'what will be will be' moment and a way of letting go of any fight. There was no point fighting, or trying to figure it all out. All that was making it worse.

Once I understood this, everything started to become clearer. Acceptance doesn't cure you, but neither does it allow anxiety and OCD to grow any further. You will still feel anxiety but as Lauren has demonstrated, this decreases by increments over time. This is because you're no longer feeding it with fight. You aren't fighting, you aren't reassuring – you're just accepting what is, in all its various forms.

A word of warning, though: don't fall into the trap of using the concept of 'acceptance' as a safety behaviour. Don't say to yourself, 'I'm accepting, I'm accepting' because that will become a compulsion. Remember when I kept telling myself that it was all 'just fear'? That worked for a while until the day it didn't, and I had what is best described as a nervous breakdown as a result. True acceptance is NOT telling yourself that it's acceptance. It's about feeling it, just letting it be there, for however long it wants to stay.

Remember to truly and honestly accept your state of mind; don't fall into the trap of just saying the words. Simply telling yourself that you accept your state of mind is NOT true acceptance. It may make you feel a bit better for a little while, but be careful, as saying it to yourself over and over again is nothing more than reassurance which can become a compulsion in itself. Remember Lauren's advice, which is to be compassionate to yourself – you can achieve this by allowing your mind to accept what it is, have the courage to let the thoughts, emotions and sensations be there and for you to do absolutely nothing with them while you endeavour to go about your day.

When you begin this process of true and absolute acceptance of your state of mind then you are no longer in negotiation with your thoughts, urges, emotions and fears and therefore you are no longer feeding the anxiety. It will, of course, still hang around – it's not going to sulk off that easily! It's been so used to you feeding it and getting its way whenever it wants to, due to your actions of questioning it, negotiating with it and fighting it. Therefore, let it hang around as much as it wants, but like anything in life, when you stop feeding it or cut off its fuel supply it will try and persevere, but eventually it will stop working.

In my view, acceptance is the first platform to recovery from anxiety. If you carry this out truthfully and honestly to yourself, you will begin to cull any further growth in the unwanted anxiety and will eventually start to see the results for yourself first hand.

WHAT DOES TRUE ACCEPTANCE FEEL LIKE?

When you first take the leap of faith into acceptance, it can be very scary. It feels really uncomfortable and even stressful. This will almost feel counter-productive in dealing with your anxiety as you will feel an initial further spike in your anxiety levels. For the first time in your life you are going to let your guard down, give up the fight and simply allow your thoughts and sensations which are fuelling your anxious state of mind to do and say what they want. How scary, right? You are going into the unknown! You are feeling the anxiety without fighting it, which initially makes you feel on edge. It makes you very uncomfortable; it will do its best to tempt you and get you to go through things in your mind just one more time, just so it feels right.

Don't fall for this!

Don't negotiate with the temptation of thinking it through. Take the leap and let all the feelings which are fuelling your anxiety be there in all their glory.

As the acceptance process takes hold, it becomes liberating. When I first truly started to have faith in myself to accept my state of mind and not fight or negotiate with my intrusive thoughts, my confidence began to grow each day and my internal fear, instigated by unwanted and intrusive thoughts which had tormented me all my life, began to naturally subside as each day and week passed. If you truly embrace an absolute acceptance of your current mental health issues, you will have taken a huge step towards your recovery.

What I have come to realise is that anxiety-based mental health issues are not our intrusive and unwanted thoughts themselves. All human beings on this planet have these kinds of thoughts every single day. We can't stop or control any of the 50,000 to 70,000 thoughts that instantaneously pop into our minds each day and nor would we want to. Our thoughts allow us to live, evolve and aspire. However, mental health issues and conditions that are found in sufferers like me are in fact created and exacerbated by our reactions, interpretations and meanings that we give to these unwanted thoughts. It's not the thought itself that causes the damage, it's the meaning we give it.

Unconditional ACCEPTANCE of your intrusive thoughts and letting them simply be there without giving them any interaction lays the perfect platform for recovery.

I'd say it took me about a month to come to terms with what acceptance is. After that point, it started to come into my life naturally. That was the stage when I knew I was accepting things, but wasn't analysing why and how I was. All thoughts, whether good or bad, come from the same place in the brain. I accept the good thoughts and the nice emotions which are associated with them. By approaching my unwanted and intrusive thoughts exactly the same way, they started to come and go just as easily as my good thoughts did. It felt incredibly liberating. Nothing could harm me, because I didn't care whether it did or it didn't. For the first time in my life, no matter what was being thrown at me, my reaction was simply 'Let it go'. I wasn't even trying to figure it out. And yes, I began to feel better, and ready to start the next stage of my recovery, which was all about **embracing** anxiety, hugging it close to me, inviting it to come towards me, and going towards it. Read on, and find out how to **embrace** your anxiety as I did, thereby reducing it to an insignificant little nothing, a minor inconvenience.

SECTION 2

EMBRACE

Part A: Lauren: Now we have understood and **accepted** our anxiety problem, what are we going to do about it? We've seen how OCD and anxiety is fuelled, and how it goes round in a vicious cycle, even as we carry out common, creative and sometimes weird strategies to avoid it. As we know, these strategies actually keep the problem going.

So, logically, the way to break the cycle is not to avoid but to **embrace** unhelpful thoughts, seeing them for what they are. We need to explore the way you're interpreting your trigger (i.e. the external event or unhelpful thought) to see if:

a) the threat you're perceiving is really probable or likely to be true,

and

b) whether there are any other explanations for it.

As we know, in life there are almost always two sides to every story. So let's say there is another story to explain your anxiety and obsessions. We'll call this the '**Two Hands Theory**'. As an example, let's look at Adam's fear of harming someone.

On the One Hand, his OCD told him he was an actual danger to other people.

BUT ...

On the Other Hand, he might also have recognised that his problem was that he was a sensitive, caring person who was **worried** about being a danger to other people rather than being an actual danger.

Having read Adam's story, which of the '**Two Hands**' explanations do you think is actually true? If you guessed it was the '**Other Hand**', you're absolutely correct.

> Adam's problem wasn't that he was an actual danger to people; it was that he WORRIED about being a danger to them.

Of course, this might seem like an easy conclusion to come to, but it isn't. Adam was convinced he was a danger to others; he truly felt that way and went to extreme lengths to avoid such feelings. So to help him decide which of the '**Two Hands**' explanations was true, I had to let him weigh up the evidence for himself. Had he ever attacked anyone? Had he made a plan to attack anyone? Had he been diagnosed with psychopathic tendencies? Did he carry a weapon around with the intent to harm someone? Did he enjoy these thoughts of harming people? The answer to each and every one of these questions was a resounding 'NO'. There was no evidence that Adam was a danger to other people, although we can't predict the future and I couldn't guarantee 100 per cent that Adam wouldn't become a danger at some time. However, from what we knew it was highly unlikely as there was no evidence of this happening in the past and no evidence it was likely to happen.

Looking at another example, let's say you are worried about making presentations at work to your colleagues in case you make a mistake and look like you don't know what you are talking about, so you avoid doing so at all cost (including potential to progress in the role!). Using the **Two Hands Theory**, we can look at this in the same way.

On the One Hand, your anxiety is telling you that you are going to make a mistake and everyone will think that you can't do your job properly.

BUT ...

On the Other Hand, you are worried that you will make a mistake as you like your job and it is important to you to do well at work, and you have lost confidence in yourself.

Similar to Adam's worry about harming people, this is something that has not yet happened! Even if you have made a mistake in the past during a presentation, it does not mean you will make a mistake in the future. I cannot guarantee that you will not make a mistake during a presentation in the future, but I can guarantee that the more you avoid giving a presentation, the more you will worry about it and suffer the consequences of anxiety. The problem is not one of making mistakes, it is one of *worrying* about making a mistake.

> **I can't guarantee that what you're worried about won't happen in the future, but it is so unlikely that it's not worth living your life restricted by the possibility.**

When you read this you will no doubt feel very uncomfortable. That's OK – I would expect that. What you want is a 100 per cent guarantee that what you are worried about won't happen. No one can give you this. This is a common thinking problem in anxiety and obsessional problems; **Guarantees for the Future**, and it was mentioned in the previous section. Adam was **Catastrophising** – thinking the worst thing would be that he would harm someone – he had a **Magnified Sense of Duty** (believing he was responsible for making sure this didn't happen) and wanted a **Guarantee for the Future** that this would not happen. So you can see he had a number of unhelpful thinking problems in play here.

The person worrying about making a mistake in their work presentation also has a number of thinking problems. They are **Catastrophising** by thinking that the worst outcome will happen, seeking a **Guarantee for the Future** that they wouldn't make a mistake, and also **Overestimating the likelihood** that they would make a mistake. They are also **Mind reading** by thinking that they know what their colleagues would think if they did make a mistake.

In addition, what both Adam and the person worried about the work presentation did not like, was the feeling of **Not Knowing** what was going to happen. This can also be described as an **Intolerance of Uncertainty** – finding it very difficult to tolerate the feeling of being unsure. In fact, in all anxiety and obsessional problems you will find that people suffer from an **Intolerance of Uncertainty**. This feels very uncomfortable and people spend their time trying to perform rituals, compulsions and safety behaviours to reduce any uncertainty. In reality, of course, there is nothing certain about life apart from death. But in anxiety disorders people apply an **All-or-Nothing** thinking approach and try and force situations to fit into a '100 per cent certain' box, as in 'I need to be 100 per cent certain this thing will not happen', or they decide it is 'intolerable' to be uncertain so must continually try and aim for 100 per cent certainty.

SITUATION: 'I must be 100 per cent certain this bad thing will not happen in the future'

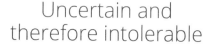

 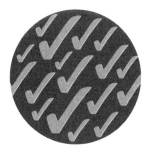

Figure 7: Seeking total certainty in an all-or-nothing approach.

The problem with this approach is that as there is no certainty to anything in life, it always ends up in the 'intolerable – must keep trying' box. If we think about this in a tick-box approach, as shown above in Figure 7, Adam was only giving himself two options – that he had to be 100 per cent certain that he wasn't going to hurt someone, or it wasn't good enough and he had to work harder to get to tick the '100 per cent certainty' box. This is an impossible dilemma – your goal of 100 per cent certainty doesn't exist, yet you are striving for a non-existent goal. You only end up in the 'intolerable – must keep trying for certainty' box.

A more helpful approach is to see this on a continuum or sliding scale and ask yourself to rate things on a confidence approach. For example, at the beginning of treatment Adam may only be 60 per cent confident that he would not hurt someone because he is consumed by doubt, but that still means he can see it is not a given fact that he will harm someone, and it is easier to tolerate being unsure if you are partly confident that the bad thing won't happen. If you rate yourself on this scale at different points of the day or stages of treatment, you will move up and down the continuum. This shows that we have more flexibility in the way we think about things. At the end of treatment Adam may be 99.5 per cent confident that he will not harm someone, and there is still that 0.5 per cent doubt, but this feels much better. There may be days where he is only 75 per cent confident, but that also feels better than the doubt he had at the beginning of treatment.

'How confident am I that I won't hurt someone?'

New, more flexible approach

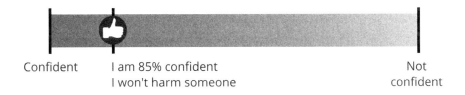

Figure 8: A more flexible approach.

In the case of the person worried about giving a presentation at work, the continuum is likely to look like:

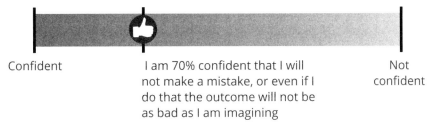

Figure 9: Another example of adopting a more flexible approach.

After introducing a sliding scale, I then put another set of questions to Adam. Did the thought of harming people disturb and upset him? Did he go to extreme lengths to avoid knives, and anything else that could be considered a weapon? Did he avoid the news, and TV programmes that contained violence? The answer to each question was, of course, a 'YES'.

So although it seemed Adam's problem was one of him being **worried** that he was going to hurt someone, in fact he was living like he *was* a dangerous person. Not just that he worried about it. Similarly, the person who is worried about the work presentation is living like it is predetermined that they will make a mistake.

If we examine your problem on the **'Two Hands'** basis, and subject it to rigorous questioning, we can see another explanation evolving for your reaction to the trigger. Let's have a look at another scenario and subject it to the same 'Two Hands' test.

Let's say your anxiety is based around leaving water running in the house. You can't go out without checking all the taps are turned off (and you're turning them off so tightly that other people in the house can't turn them back on easily!). You're anxious about this because you've read in the paper about a ceiling collapsing in a house as a result of a flooded bathroom. Because you think you're careless, you believe this could happen to you.

Let's look at the evidence for the **One Hand.** This viewpoint suggests that I am careless and will flood that house and cause immense damage. Therefore, I will try to ensure that this does not happen, hence my behaviour of checking and turning taps off.

Ask yourself: Where did I hear about this? Was it just the one incident, or do I read about it every day? Were there any other circumstances? Has it happened to me before? And if it has, what was the outcome? Has it happened to anyone I know? Is there any evidence for this viewpoint? How many houses have I flooded before?

If you answer these truthfully, you'll probably realise that such an incident is pretty rare, and the odds of it happening to you are very small. And, if you have ever left taps on or dripping, the consequences were likely not as bad as you imagined them to be. Overall, there is very little solid evidence for this viewpoint.

But you are living like it is an imminent possibility.

OK, let's look at the **Other Hand**. This viewpoint suggests that I believe it's important to be careful and take care of my home, and I *WORRY* that something bad will happen. Ask yourself: Am I worrying about this? Do I feel anxious in my body? Do I worry too much? Have I worried about other things that never happened? Will turning the tap off tightly or checking it multiple times guarantee 100 per cent that my ceiling won't fall in because of a flood?

If you answer these truthfully you'll probably realise that your anxiety is based on the **worry** of this happening, rather than it actually happening. In life, we can't guarantee that anything won't happen to us. The likelihood of your ceiling falling in is so small that it is insignificant, and even though your anxiety is trying to tell you it is a real possibility, it isn't worth living your life as though it will happen. And even in the very unlikely scenario it does, it will be very inconvenient for a while, but it will pass.

The difficulty most people have with the idea that the problem is not real or likely is that it means that they can't do anything about it. If you actually knew that the house was going to flood at some point in the future, then you would feel better because you could do something about it now. If you knew that you were going to make a mistake in your work presentation, you could practice it excessively and to the exclusion of other work or leisure activities. This is the thinking problem we call **Perceived Control** – you think you might be able to control but in reality you cannot. But if the problem is that you are worrying about flooding, it's difficult because you can't actually do anything to stop something what might or might not happen from happening. You are left with the feelings of anxiety and uncertainty, which you don't like, and these are not nice. But we can cope with these feelings, which we will look at further on in the PTT approach.

So while the reality of the situation can be proven, your worries still feel true. Employing the **Two Hands Theory** is a great way of examining the evidence.

Below is a box, using the **Two Hands Theory**, write down the trigger for your anxiety and list the evidence for it actually happening. To help you, there are some examples of completed forms on the following pages.

On the 'One Hand' my problem is ...

_____

_____

_____

What ways am I living my life because of this: (i.e. what am I doing to make sure it doesn't happen, and what will I need to do in the future to continue to prevent it coming true?)

_____

_____

_____

Evidence for this position being true:

_____

_____

_____

_____

_____

_____

_____

_____

_____

On this side, list the evidence against, taking worry itself into consideration. Also write down how your life might look if it was a worry-based problem.

On the 'Other Hand' my problem is that I *worry* that ...

_____

_____

Ways I could live my life if this was only a worry problem rather than it being real:

_____

_____

Evidence for this position being true:

_____

_____

_____

_____

_____

_____

_____

Based on the evidence, which position do you think is more likely to be true?

Table 9: On the One Hand vs. On the Other Hand.

Now ask yourself: If I was in a Court of Law judging this evidence, which position is the strongest? What would the verdict be – one of imminent danger happening or one of worrying about it happening?

Let's look at this again, with reference to Adam's worry about harming someone.

On the 'One Hand' my problem is that I obviously **want** to strangle or stab someone because I have had this thought, and it is only a matter of time until I do.

What ways am I making sure that this doesn't come true, and what else do I need to be doing to make sure it doesn't come true:
- Carrying handcuffs
- Keeping my hands in my pockets
- Avoiding all sharp objects
- Eating with hands and never using utensils

In the future I will need to:
- Avoid being alone with people
- Actually wear handcuffs
- Wear a straitjacket
- Never attend a meal out or at someone's house
- Hand myself in to the police – just to be sure
- Commit myself to a mental institution – just to be sure

Evidence for this position being true:
- Well, I had the thought so it must mean that I want to do it, deep down in my subconscious

On the 'Other Hand' my problem is that I **worry** that I might want to hurt someone because I have had this unpleasant thought and I've **lost confidence** that I am able to control my behaviour.

If this position is true, what do I need to be doing:

- I need to stop worrying, build up my confidence in myself and live life free of these restrictions

Evidence for this position being true:

- I have never acted on this thought
- I have never harmed anyone
- I have had unpleasant thoughts before and never acted on them
- Everyone has unpleasant thoughts
- No one else who knows me is worried about me acting on this thought, even when I tell them about my thoughts
- I feel anxious when I have this thought, which suggests it is an anxiety/worry problem
- I have a history of having unpleasant thoughts, but nothing bad has happened from having these thoughts
- Just because I had a thought it does not make it true (for example thinking I will win the lottery, or thinking something unpleasant will happen such as a car accident)

Based on the evidence, which position do you think is more likely to be true?

Table 10: Example of a completed form showing On the One Hand vs. On the Other Hand.

Table 11: *Another example of a completed form showing On the One Hand vs. On the Other Hand.*

On the 'One Hand' my problem is that I will make a mistake in my presentation at work and everyone will think that I am not competent to do my job.

What ways am I making sure that this doesn't come true, and what else do I need to be doing to make sure it doesn't come true:
- Avoiding presentations
- If I have to speak up or present my work, I practise it over and over and over again
- Making sure that I am over prepared for any meeting in case I am asked about my work

Evidence for this position being true:
- Well, I once made a mistake during a course presentation at university and felt mortified

On the 'Other Hand' my problem is that I **worry** I'll make a mistake in my work presentation and I **worry** that it means people will think I am not competent to do my job, I've **lost confidence** in myself.

If this position is true, what do I need to be doing:
- I need to stop worrying, build up my confidence in myself and be more relaxed in my approach to meetings
- I can stop practising any presentation to the exclusion of other activities

Evidence for this position being true:
- It hasn't happened yet! I can't predict the future
- Even in the past when I made a mistake in a presentation, some people said afterwards they didn't even notice
- Despite making a mistake, I still got a good grade for a piece of work
- I have had to speak at a lot of meetings, and previously have made work presentations, and have not made any big mistakes
- Mistakes are normal! Everyone makes them
- Other people have made mistakes and I don't think less of them or that they are not competent to do their job
- I don't know what other people are thinking! I am not privy to their thoughts
- I feel anxious when I think about doing presentations, which suggests it is an anxiety/worry problem

Based on the evidence, which position do you think is more likely to be true?

WORRY

Hopefully now you're beginning to see that the problem is one of interpretation, not of reality itself. It is an emotional problem, and what you've been doing so far is pushing away or avoiding unpleasant thoughts because you don't like the feeling of anxiety they are giving you. But remember: you are not wholly responsible for anything. There are things beyond your control, and if you try to take 100 per cent responsibility for everything (**Magnified Duty**) by doing everything in your power not to let bad things happen, you will feel anxious, drained and incapable of living your life as you want to. You now know that your responses so far have been fuelling these feelings. And please note that I haven't told you to simply 'stop worrying'! Telling yourself that is another way of avoiding the feelings of anxiety – exactly like Adam's 'just fear' mantra. Worries might not be based in reality, but they certainly feel real and telling someone with chronic worry to stop worrying is like asking them to stop breathing!

So how do we manage our worry, by seeing it for what it is and reducing its ability to interfere in our daily lives? The answer is that, rather than running away and avoiding it, we have to go right up to it and embrace it. As Adam would say, we have to 'bring it on'. Even me just saying that will probably stir feelings of anxiety within you but please keep reading and following the PTT approach. Embracing the trigger which is prompting your anxiety, again and again, is the only way to make it shrink into the shadows and disappear altogether. Part B of this section will feel challenging and is indeed very challenging, but please stay with us. This part of the approach will quite possibly be the one which changes your life forever.

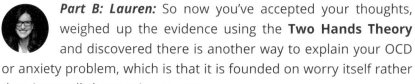 ***Part B: Lauren:*** So now you've accepted your thoughts, weighed up the evidence using the **Two Hands Theory** and discovered there is another way to explain your OCD or anxiety problem, which is that it is founded on worry itself rather than it actually happening to you.

But despite that, you still feel bad. Of course you do! OCD and anxiety aren't going to give up that easily. Just because you've discovered their nasty little secret doesn't mean they'll automatically slink away. In fact, like Adam, if you start telling yourself that it's 'just fear' or 'just worry', you're going to start worrying about the worry itself, and so the vicious cycle of anxiety will keep on spinning.

As I said at the end of Part A, the way to overcome this – the **ONLY** way – is to pull the trigger: go towards whatever it is that is causing your worry and embrace it. The more you do this, the easier it will be to '**habituate**' yourself to the thing or thought that prompts your anxiety, until you get to the point where this trigger is no longer one of fear – it has become normal.

Now, the paragraph above runs counter to everything you've attempted so far to control your anxiety problem. You've run away from it, or pushed it aside using rituals, safety behaviours or avoidance strategies. It's felt better for a while, but it hasn't gone away totally; if anything, it has eventually become worse. And even though you now know there is another explanation for your OCD and anxiety, you still feel jittery every time you think about it.

Perhaps you're asking yourself, '**What if**?' What if it is the '**One Hand**' explanation which is true, as opposed to the '**Other Hand**', and the thing you are anxious about DOES come true? The big dog bites you, the ceiling falls in, you attack someone in the street – what if, what if, what if?

Well, if you're asking yourself 'What if?', please be assured that it is a perfectly normal thing to ask. I've yet to meet anyone in therapy with OCD or anxiety who doesn't have doubts about the process, especially around exposure. 'There's no way I can do THAT!' people tell me. 'THAT'S the very thing which is causing all this!' Having doubts is fine. You've lived so long with OCD and anxiety, you're bound to feel nervous as we go into this stage of the PTT approach. But as I always say – stay with me. If you do, I promise your life will improve.

So let's look at a typical habituation model. To explain this, I've drawn two graphs on the following page. The first shows what happens when you come up against your trigger and you make your anxiety go away, using your tried-and-tested methods of avoidance and safety behaviours:

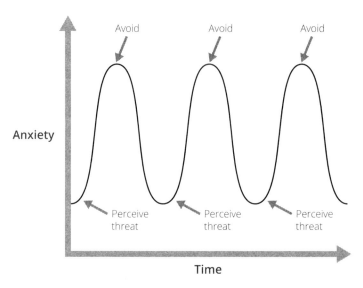

Figure 10: *Avoidance of threat.*

In this first graph, we see that every time you detect a threat your anxiety level shoots up until you carry out your safety behaviour. Then it drops back down. Unfortunately, the next time your anxiety is triggered up it goes again, until you perform your safety behaviour and it brings the anxiety back down. And so on and so on, meaning that nothing is being done to reduce the anxiety permanently.

This second graph shows what happens when you don't avoid your trigger, but embrace and expose yourself to it:

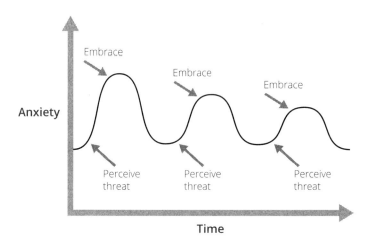

Figure 11: *Exposure to threat/habituation of anxiety.*

What we're now seeing is that if you embrace/expose yourself to the threat, over time it decreases. For example, say you have a phobia around dogs, and every time you see one your anxiety shoots up. In normal circumstances you'd run away to counteract the fear – but next time you see a dog the same thing happens again. However, if we're working around your dog phobia and I bring a dog to our next session and you don't avoid the situation and stay in the room, you're going to feel very uncomfortable – but I can guarantee that the next time I bring the dog in, you will still feel uncomfortable, but slightly less so. That's because you're now **habituating** to the threat (the dog), and each time I bring him in your anxiety will eventually lessen and over time will reduce much quicker. Your body and brain start to learn that the threat is not as bad as you thought, and that you survived. This works only as long as you are not doing an avoidance or neutralising behaviour, such as calming yourself down by saying something in your head or by shutting your eyes, for example.

'OK,' I hear you say, 'but I don't want to go near that dog in the first place, never mind be in the same room as it.' That's understandable; whatever your trigger is, the anxiety around it has been troubling you for a long time and it feels very strange and uncomfortable to suddenly stand up to it, and see it for what it is.

Let's use an analogy to make this part of the process feel easier. Two lumberjacks employ a school-leaver to work with them in the forest. On his first day they decide to play a prank on him by telling him to hold up a large, low-hanging branch of a tree which, they explain, is in danger of falling down because it is so old. They say that they will come back with their tools to prune the smaller branches on the branch so it does not fall off the tree. Then they walk off and leave him standing alone, supporting the branch. A walker comes along and asks the boy why he's propping up the branch.

'Because it will fall down otherwise,' he replies.

'How do you know?' the walker asks.

'Because that's what I've been told.'

Instead of laughing at him and carrying on, the walker suggests he takes **One Hand** away from the branch. He's not keen, because he's been told to hold it up and he doesn't want to lose his job on the first day.

Neither does he want the branch to fall on his head. However, he takes the plunge and removes **One Hand**, albeit tentatively. The branch doesn't move.

'OK,' says the walker, 'why don't you take your other hand away now?'

'No way,' replies the boy. 'This might be the hand that stops the whole thing crashing down.'

'On the other hand,' replies the walker, 'that might not happen at all. It might just be that you're worried it will happen. Maybe you should try it and see?'

Gingerly, the boy removes the other hand. The tree remains as steady as it has done for the past 200 years. The boy looks at it.

'It's old,' he said. 'It could still just fall down.'

'In that case,' says the walker, 'why don't you swing on the branch?'

The boy is very nervous. Of course he is – instead of supporting the branch he is now going to do the opposite and try to make it fall down! He grabs the branch with both hands and begins to swing. Surprise, surprise – nothing happens!!

The lesson is that you never know until you try, and it's the same with anxiety. You just have to see what happens – and as we've said, there are no guarantees in life other than death. You have to put up with some uncertainty in life. So what's stopping you from at least giving it a go? You will still feel anxious, unsure and worried, but less so each time.

So what I'm asking you to do is conduct a series of experiments around your anxiety. I want you to encounter the thing you fear or the thought that is troubling you. Essentially I want you to swing from that branch like the lumberjack's assistant. I want you to leave the house with the lights on or the tap dripping. I want you to be in a place full of strangers you feel you might harm. You might want to do this alone – in fact, it can be better if you do it alone, as having someone with you could be a kind of safety behaviour. However, you might want to tell a close friend or relative that you're carrying out an experiment so that they can check in with you after you've completed it.

Sharing after the event is very useful. And, as a therapist, I will always participate in the early experiments too. For example, if I ask someone with anxiety over contamination to lick their shoe, I will do this with them. If I ask someone to wish harm on their family, I will do this too. If someone is worried about complaining about a product they have bought, I will complain first. If someone is worried they will harm someone by pushing them down the stairs, I will stand at the edge of the top of the stairs and make them put pressure on my back. If someone is worried about big dogs, I will go up to a dog in the park and ask to stroke it. If someone is worried they will jump off a bridge, I will sit on the ledge swinging my legs with them. If someone is worried that people look at them because they 'look' weird or strange, I will smear dirt on my face and walk down the busy streets or go into a shop to buy something.

Before you set out on your experiment (which I will assist you with in Part C), please have a look at the boxes on the following page and fill in the second one. I want you to write what you intend to do during your experiment and, bearing in mind the **Two Hands Theory**, note down what the **One Hand** is telling you before you set out, i.e. how thinking about doing this experiment is affecting you, and what your anxiety is telling you might happen. Then write down the other explanation for your problem, i.e. what the **Other Hand** is telling you. Be honest, and after you've done it, turn to Part C.

First, here's a couple of examples:

My experiment is to ...	My experiment is to ...
• Walk to the other side of the bridge	• Walk in the park close to where I see everyone walking their dogs
On the 'one hand' my OCD/anxiety says ...	**On the 'One Hand' my OCD/anxiety says ...**
• That I will jump off this bridge because I'm mentally unwell	• That a dog will break free from their lead and attack me
On the 'Other Hand' ...	**On the 'Other Hand' ...**
• My worry problem is telling me that I will be anxious and feel really uncomfortable, but I am not likely to throw myself off the bridge	• My worry problem is telling me that I will be anxious and feel really uncomfortable, but I am not likely to be attacked by a dog

Table 12: *Examples of setting experiments.*

Now fill in the box below:

My experiment is to ...

On the 'One Hand' my OCD/anxiety says ...

On the 'Other Hand' ...

Table 13: *Setting my own experiment.*

Part C: Lauren: Now you are ready to walk out of the door, and into a realm where there are people, situations and events which will activate your trigger. It feels scary, but you now know there is another explanation for your OCD and anxiety – one that is founded on worry itself.

In Part B you filled in the box which asked you how thinking about the experiment made you feel, and what your anxiety is telling you might happen. You think you know how you feel and what might happen – so let's go and try it out!!

In the first instance I'm going to imagine that your problem is around a fear of crossing bridges, as in the box above. For years, your anxiety has told you that if you walk over a bridge, you will throw yourself from it into the water or onto the railway line below. It's never happened to you, or anyone you know, but you've heard of such things happening and read about it in the paper. So it has happened in the past, and even though the **Two Hands Theory** has made you realise that it is your fear about what might happen that is far outstripping reality, you're still scared. So let's **embrace** that fear right now.

Let me walk with you to the beginning of that bridge. On the way we will chat normally, even though you're visibly frightened. As we turn the corner the beginning of the bridge comes into view. People are walking over it, just as they do every day. They think nothing of it. You, however, are experiencing the physiological symptoms connected with the vicious cycle of anxiety. You feel sweaty and sick, your breathing has become shallow. You think that you cannot do this. But we will keep walking, right up to the beginning of the bridge.

As people jostle past us, on their way to work or to the shops, we stop. You look at me, and tell me you can't cross. Fine. I would never force you to do something you don't want to do. I will explain, however, that it is your anxiety and fear that is stopping you from taking this step. It is not that you will throw yourself off. It is your worry that you will. I will tell you that you can take the first steps, so you walk ahead and onto the bridge.

What happens next? That's up to you! Let's say you walked 10 yards, paused, and came back. That's OK. Although you didn't go as far as we might have wanted, and your anxiety level is off the scale, you walked 10 yards – **and nothing happened to you**. You survived. You didn't throw yourself into the water and drown.

You pulled your Trigger. You faced and embraced your biggest fear, and you were not annihilated.

Let's go home now, and have a think about what happened. Pat yourself on the back for what you did, but don't reassure yourself that now you've done it once, you don't ever have to do it again. You need to do this time and time again, and push yourself each time to walk further over the bridge, until you have crossed the full length of it, to **habituate** yourself to it. If we recall the graph in the previous chapter, the next time you attempt to cross the bridge you will still feel anxious, but not with the same intensity as the first time.

Notice that I didn't push you to cross the bridge. This is an experiment in habituation, NOT a challenge to see if you can do the whole thing in one go. I would rather we start to try it out, step by step. For example, if you fear that leaving the tap dripping in the bathroom will lead to a flood, I will first ask you to turn the tap on so it is dripping steadily, and then go out of the house for ten minutes, then come back and see if what you feared has come true. If you fear you will harm people, I might ask you to place a pair of scissors in your pocket, catch a crowded bus and get off at the next stop. The next time, you can leave the tap dripping for fifteen minutes or travel a couple more stops. So you build up your exposure to the fear, experiencing each one as a progression towards a time when you are no longer having such fearful reactions. My approach is to get you to acknowledge that some things feel scarier than others and I won't ask you to do the scariest thing at the moment – but it will happen sooner than you think. Even so, take each day at a time.

Using another example, let's say that you are scared of dogs and worried about being attacked by a dog. Your first experiment might be to just walk to the park close to the dog walking enclosure. As you have avoided going to parks for a long time in case there were dogs there, this is going to be challenging for you. But you have recognised that you have a worry based problem and it is highly unlikely that a dog will attack you. Despite feeling very anxious, you manage to complete your experiment, and whilst walking around you feel on edge and on guard for any dogs, but no dog comes close to you!

It was unpleasant and scary, but you did it and returned home safe! If you repeat this same experiment over the next few times, you will find that you habituate and each time you do the experiment you will feel less anxious.

In a similar vein, the person worried about the work presentation might plan to do a 5 minute presentation on some training they have attended in the next team meeting. Again, this will be scary and, without over preparing or excessive practising, they manage to do the presentation. They find they either make no mistakes, or if they made one, it was minor and no one seemed bothered by it! So next week they agree to do a follow up presentation on another topic. Each time they do an experiment they will become less anxious and are building up confidence in their presenting abilities.

OK, so we got to the bridge and you walked 10 yards. Remembering this is a metaphor, how did it feel when you did your own experiment?

Have a look at the boxes on the next page, read the examples first and then fill in your own conclusions:

Table 14: *Examples of completed experiments and how to build upon them.*

Experiment of walking across the bridge

Did the 'One Hand' prediction come true?
- No.

How did you feel?
- Very anxious that I would harm myself, but relieved it didn't happen.

If the 'Other Hand' position that you have a worry-based problem that causes you to feel anxious is true, what does this mean for you now?
- I should stop worrying!

What do you conclude from this experiment?
- That I need to work on worry but I am unlikely to throw myself off a bridge.

What is my anxiety problem or OCD trying to tell me now?
- That even if it is worry, how do I know I won't harm myself in some other way such as jumping in front of a train?

How can I challenge this with an experiment?
- Visit a train station and stand on the platform closer to the edge than feels comfortable.

Experiment of walking in the park around dogs

Did the 'One Hand' prediction come true?
- No.

How did you feel?
- Very anxious that I would be attacked by a dog and relieved it didn't happen.

If the 'Other Hand' position is that you have a worry-based problem that causes you to feel anxious is true, what does this mean for you now?
- I should stop worrying!

What do you conclude from this experiment?
- That I need to work on worry but it is very unlikely that a dog is going to attack me.

What is my anxiety problem trying to tell me now?
- That even if it is worry, how do I know that I won't be attacked by a dog in the future when I go to a different park?

How can I challenge this with an experiment?
- Visit different parks and walk around them, especially in the morning or evening when people are likely to be walking their dogs.

Experiment of giving a presentation at work

Did the 'One Hand' prediction come true?
- No.

How did you feel?
- Very anxious that I would make a mistake during the presentation and that people would notice and think I am not fit to do my job.

If the 'Other Hand' position is that you have a worry-based problem that causes you to feel anxious is true, what does this mean for you now?
- I should stop worrying!

What do you conclude from this experiment?
- That I can do presentations despite feeling anxious, and that I won't necessarily make a mistake.

What is my anxiety problem trying to tell me now?
- I might make a mistake next time I do an experiment.

How can I challenge this with an experiment?
- Volunteer to do more presentations, and even make a small mistake on purpose and see what happens.

Now fill in this box with your own experience:

Did the 'One Hand' prediction come true?

_____

How did you feel?

_____

_____

If the 'Other Hand' position is that you have a worry-based problem that causes you to feel anxious is true, what does this mean for you now?

_____

_____

What do you conclude from this experiment?

_____

_____

What is my anxiety problem or OCD trying to tell me now?

_____

_____

_____

How can I challenge this with an experiment?

_____

_____

_____

Table 15: _Analysing the outcome of the experiment._

If you've answered honestly, hopefully you'll have acknowledged that while you felt fearful, the **One Hand** prediction you've always told yourself will happen, hasn't happened. And hopefully you will conclude that worry is the driver of your OCD and anxiety.

Above all, what I really hope is that you will continue the experiment, no matter how scary it felt the first time. Walk over that bridge, without me, again and again and again. Visit more parks, and even visit a kennel. Continue to volunteer to do more work presentations. The more you **EMBRACE** your fears, the more times you face them – and face them down – the quicker your anxiety will reduce. Remember *Figure 11: Exposure to threat/habituation of anxiety,* in the last chapter, and each time you do an experiment notice how long it took you for your anxiety levels to return to normal. That way, you will be able to see it reduce. And also take each day as it comes. There may be days when you have worries about the effectiveness of the experiments, and whether you're actually getting better at all. As I've said before – this is normal. If you are a person who doesn't have any doubts, it's very unlikely you would be reading this book and PTT approach in the first place!

The more you become attuned to the idea of experiments, the more you can put yourself in a position where you can take on more complicated and/or challenging ones. If, for example, you're worried that you might be a paedophile because you've had an intrusive thought about a child (as I've said, by no means uncommon these days), you could walk past schools at lunchtime or spend twenty minutes or so in a toy shop. This will feel really uncomfortable at first, but stay with it – in time, your anxiety will reduce. I've worked with people who worry that others think they are a paedophile, so I get them to shout 'I am a paedophile!' twenty times over and record it on their phone and write it on a note and put it in their pocket to keep there for a week. Then I ask them to play the recording to themselves several times a day. Again, that's very uncomfortable but it works.

Other examples could be that if you're worried that you're not paying attention because of your OCD – and, for example, if you frequently need to drive your children around and worry that you might crash, and therefore you avoid driving your children around

– then you need to carry out an activity that requires such attention, when you are feeling anxious, such as going for a short drive with someone. If your obsession is around Social Services taking your children away because they know you worry about harming them, then tell your medical practitioner or another health professional about your anxieties. If you are worried about traveling on airplanes, book and take a very short flight. If you are worried about getting food poisoning after eating seafood, make sure you eat some shrimp.

So you need to work out where your anxiety is based and go right to the source. It's not always easy – it rarely is – but the more you habituate to it, the quicker you will recover.

Another example – you might have OCD and anxiety around a religious-based fear of saying something that would offend a deity. Religious-themed OCD is very common, but again very frightening for people for whom the observance of their religion is very important. But remember, **OCD attacks the most important things to us!** If religion wasn't important to you, then it would be very unlikely that you would have OCD about religion. Religious OCD can be very paralysing for people who expect that their God(s) or deities will punish them or their families for the thoughts they're having. But let's look at this situation using the Two Hands Theory. You may think on the **One Hand** that having these thoughts means that 'I am a bad person and my God(s) will punish me for having these thoughts in the afterlife.' Now that is a difficult position to disprove, and we can't disprove it, but as you recall, the way to challenge OCD is not to disprove it. In fact, in trying to disprove the OCD, you end up feeding the OCD by creating more doubt and more worries. There are no guarantees about the future, and this also applies to religious beliefs about the future.

So maybe on the **Other Hand** you are worried about having these thoughts as your religious observance is very important to you, but having intrusions is normal and your God(s) understands that it is just a worry problem. I have spoken with various religious leaders, including Catholic priests and Muslim imams over the years, and they all accept that intrusions, however awful the content, are normal and that everyone, including themselves, have them.

If someone is having intrusive thoughts about their God(s) I would ask them to stand outside a church or equivalent religious building (or even inside) and say what the intrusions are out loud. If they are 'jumping on the branch', as in pushing back against their OCD, I may encourage them to say other inappropriate things about their God(s) or their religion, then see what happens. By doing this, you will see these thoughts for what they are – just thoughts. In no way do I want to challenge people's religious beliefs, as obviously it is very important for people to believe in and observe religion. But ask yourself, 'Would my God(s) prefer me to be anxious and feel terrible and likely avoid all religious practices in case they trigger intrusive thoughts, as can happen in religious OCD, or would my God(s) understand that I have an anxiety problem and that intrusions are normal, and would prefer me to get better from my problem and spend my time engaged in religious activities without worry?' If it is the second one, then your God(s) will understand that you need to do experiments in order to beat the OCD and anxiety and get better.

In a similar way, I have dealt with people who worry about future-based events. 'If I think this bad thought now,' they think, 'in five years' time my grandmother will die.' So there is a long gap between the intrusive thought and the perceived event taking place, and the trick is to show people that their thoughts do not contain magical powers. So perhaps I will ask the client to think something bad about me – 'Lauren, as you're going home you will fall and break your leg' – and get them to say this out loud, almost as a curse. Once I'm home I will text them to say that I'm OK, or let them know whether in fact I have broken my leg! We'll keep doing this as the period of time between the 'curse' and its 'coming true' is longer and longer. Eventually, the client will realise that their thinking is not magical after all. Other future focused anxieties include worrying about things that have not happened yet, but are not contingency based so are not considered to be 'magical thinking'. For example, if you are worried about having work in the future to support your family. I cover these type of worries under the general category 'worries about the future' starting on page 167.

Also, let's look at one of the **Thinking Errors** we mentioned earlier in the PTT approach and see how we embrace them. One was **Magnified Duty** – thinking that you're responsible for everything, and doing everything you can to make sure bad things don't happen.

Now, I can tell you to embrace your fear and leave all the lights and appliances on, then go out for thirty minutes. But you might tell me, 'Hang on, I'm 100 per cent responsible for those lights. If the house catches fire and burns down, that's my responsibility and I can't handle that.'

Well, let's see. To help, let's draw a pie chart which can divide up this responsibility.[17] Say that your anxiety is based around the workplace, and each night you're the one to leave last because you feel responsible for turning everything off. But are you? How about your co-workers? What percentage of responsibility do they have for switching off their computers? How about the caretaker, or the cleaner? The Health and Safety manager, or the boss himself? Surely they all have shared responsibility for making sure the building is safe when the working day is done?

So in reality, you are only partly responsible for ensuring that things are turned off, and even within that it is a small percentage. It may FEEL that you are more responsible (see the thinking problems **Emotional Reasoning** and **Magnified Duty**) but in reality you are not. In fact, the best experiment to test this out is NOT to turn off anything, including your own computer, before leaving for the night and see what happens!

The first pie chart is how you perceive your responsibility:

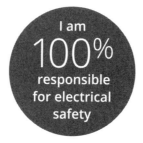

Figure 12: Responsibility pie chart: what my Anxiety/OCD is telling me.

17 Van Oppen, P. and Arntz, A. (1994). Cognitive therapy for obsessive-compulsive disorder. *Behaviour Research and Therapy*, 32(1), 79–87.

This is how responsibility is shared out in reality:

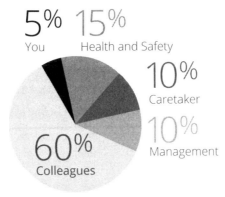

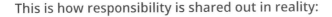

Figure 13: Responsibility pie chart: a more realistic approach.

You may experience **Magnified Duty** thinking problems in lots of situations. For example, someone who is worried about the outcome of a large work project, despite a number of other people being involved in the project. They hold themselves personally responsible for making sure the project is completed on time, even though there are a number of things outside their control. Or the person who worries whether their relatives and friends are enjoying themselves at a party. Again a number of things are outside their control, but yet they take it upon themselves to ensure everyone is having a good time! A difficult task to say the least.

Adam also had some OCD and anxiety around blinking and swallowing, and worried that he wouldn't be able to take his mind off these sensory actions, that he would always be constantly aware of these actions and would be in a permanent locked-in state of thinking about blinking and swallowing. So I made him sit in front of a mirror and watch himself as he did both, and he had to only think about blinking and swallowing for ten minutes at a time. Eventually it became hard for him to maintain that concentration and he realised that **trying not to think about it** was what was causing the problem, not the action itself. I also used to text him at random times to ask him whether he was blinking or swallowing – by doing this it reminded him of the action, forcing him to think about it, become anxious and by doing so habituate to the anxiety it caused, and learn to accept the thoughts as just thoughts.

Eventually, there will come a time when your anxiety is at a very low point, or has disappeared altogether. The point for Adam came when he was able to hold a knife to my neck without worrying that he was going to cause harm (to me or anyone). His worst fear was right there in front of him – he's taller and stronger than me, and he was holding a weapon – and yet he was able to do this experiment and put the knife down without experiencing the anxiety and physiological symptoms that had previously troubled him so much.

'PURE O' AND MENTAL STRATEGIES

At this point it might be useful to discuss what some people refer to as 'Pure O'. This is a common term used to describe people without observable compulsions, rituals or safety behaviours, but they have the obsessions. However, it is a bit misleading. I have yet to meet anyone with Pure O obsessions without some compulsions, as there is always a compulsion or behaviour associated with the obsessions. In the case of Pure O, the compulsions or rituals can be mental – as in, they are done in your head. That is why they are not observable and people assume that just because you aren't washing your hands all the time, or turning switches on and off etc., you don't have any rituals. These mental compulsions include mental checking, mental chanting, repeating phrases or numbers in your head, scanning yourself or your environment, arguing with yourself, trying to solve the issue, avoidance of the thoughts, and ruminating. The strategies to help with these mental compulsions are covered in the next section.

People with obsessional and anxiety problems also often suffer from **Self-Focused Attention** and **Scanning**, which means that you perceive a threat and choose to focus on it, to the exclusion of other things. You will scan the environment and yourself for any evidence of the threat and whether the threat is real. The threat, of course, might be just a thought, feeling or a situation but your OCD and anxiety is telling you that it is real. So, for example, if you have a panic attack and your heart rate increases, you perceive this as something akin to a heart attack, so you pay a lot more attention to your heart rate from then on. If your problem is that you think you're a paedophile, you will be monitoring yourself for any sexual arousal symptoms when you are around children. If you are worried that you are going mad, you will monitor yourself for any signs of madness. If the problem is that you're scanning yourself for signs of sexual arousal ... the chances are you will notice something! If you are monitoring yourself for signs of madness, you will find something unusual in your thoughts. If you are paying increased attention to your heartbeat, you will notice when it beats faster even in random situations. If you are worried that other people think you are incompetent, you will scan their responses for any sign that they think that. So you can see how self-focused attention and scanning also reinforce the problem, by making you think that what you fear is in fact true or likely to happen.

To embrace this, I'd do something a little counter-intuitive which sounds like an avoidance behaviour but isn't. If we remember the **Vicious Cycle**, we will recall that the more we give something attention, the more it has us in its grip. So my strategy would be to teach people to **shift this attention** to something external. I'd ask my client to really focus in on what they're worried or anxious about for a minute. When the time is up, I'd then ask them to look at a picture on the wall of my therapy room, and ask them to spend a minute describing it out loud in detail. They'll still be feeling anxious following the first minute's task, but this will reduce quickly as their attention shifts to something else. In fact, pretty much everyone tells me they forgot what they were thinking about before I asked them to describe the picture. I use this to show the client that the threat level has not changed, but what is different is how much attention they've been paying to it, which suggests that the amount of time we spend paying attention to these things is in fact part of the problem. It is different from an avoidance/safety behaviour (which of course would reinforce the problem) because you're actively choosing to shift your attention onto something else, not because you feel you have to. It's something you can practise anywhere, on a train or a bus, in a meeting, walking down the street etc., if you notice you're scanning yourself or the external world for threats.

Try this exercise: *Think about something unpleasant that has happened recently (argument with a loved one, work issue etc.) for thirty seconds, having set a timer on your phone or clock. After the timer goes off, shift your attention to something else in the room or environment, such as a picture or a tree, and describe it out loud in a lot of detail (this should take thirty seconds).*

What happened? How did you feel in Part I compared to Part II?

Hopefully, you will see that how much attention you pay to unpleasant thoughts helps keep them present and the cycle going, and keeps you feeling anxious and depressed.

Now repeat it, and instead of saying the second part out loud, try doing it in your head. This is a bit harder, but with practice it gets easier.

And once you've learned to shift your focus onto less threatening neutral things, you will get better at being able to do it when those pesky intrusive thoughts come into your mind. And you then can do it anywhere – on the bus, waiting for a train, while in a meeting etc.

We touched a little on **Rumination** earlier in the book. This is when you focus on bad feelings and experiences from the past (as opposed to **Worry**, which is focusing on things that might happen in the present/future). You think you should've thought this way or that, and if you'd done something differently, such a thing might never have happened. Everyone does this and it's completely normal, but it becomes a problem when we can't stop it and it affects our mood. The word 'rumination' comes from 'ruminate', which is what cows and sheep do when they chew the cud, over and over and over again. It's a great description of the process, and while you think repeated turning over of the past in your mind will solve it, in fact it just makes it worse. It's like a car going round and round a roundabout many times. You feel you're going somewhere, moving forward, but in fact you're stuck in a cycle.

The most important thing here is to recognise that getting caught up in your head is a mental compulsion. It is no different from someone concerned about contamination washing their hands multiple times. Rumination can be tricky to challenge with an experiment, but if you are able to recognise that you are getting caught up, the best exposure or experiment is to **shift your attention**, as I've described above. This will leave you feeling anxious, in the same way walking across the bridge would, because you believe that if you go over and over something in your head, then you will solve it or prevent it happening again. So shifting your attention to something else will make you feel like you are not doing the right thing (as in walking across the bridge), but believe me, it is the best thing to do. Ask yourself, how much time do I spend ruminating? And how many times have I felt better for it? I am guessing none of the time! So what is the point?

People also often ask me 'How do I know it's OCD or anxiety-based ruminating?' To start with, it doesn't matter as all rumination, whether in anxiety problems, OCD or depression, is unhelpful and does not achieve anything. But I always tell my clients, 'If it looks like, behaves like, feels like OCD or anxiety or you have had the thought "this might be OCD or anxiety" – then treat it like an anxiety or an OCD problem.' Better to err on the side of caution.

It is hard to do, I know, but practise shifting your attention from internally focusing on your thoughts or physiological sensations to something external, and it will get easier to jump out of rumination and focus on the present. You are CHOOSING not to focus on your thoughts.

This is where I often explain the difference between **Avoidance** and **Distraction**. Avoidance is a problem, as you are effectively saying 'I am not going to deal with this and will ignore it', whereas helpful distraction can be useful as you are saying 'I understand and ACCEPT that this is my OCD or anxiety and that it is just me ruminating about it, so I am going to choose to think about something else.'

OK, so you can't change the past, but you can deal with it in the present. **Worries based in the future** are different to rumination, but they are still about anxieties getting trapped in your head and going round and round.

At this point we should go into a little more detail about **worry**, as there are many people who wouldn't describe themselves as OCD sufferers, but have difficulties with anxiety that manifest themselves in worry.

A 'worrier' is another way of describing someone who gets caught up thinking about what might happen in the future, usually in a catastrophic way. They think about all the possibilities that could happen, usually negative, and subsequently find it hard to enjoy life and won't take risks in case their worries become true. A lot of people say they are worriers, but some worry more than others. These people find that worry interferes in their lives; they become caught up in unhelpful thinking about the future and all the bad things that might happen to them. For example, some of us might consider the possibility of a terrorist attack occurring while we're on vacation, but will go and enjoy the vacation anyway. Worriers who allow themselves to seriously consider such a possibility might spend the entire fortnight in their room, afraid to go out and explore, or they may even cancel their vacation altogether. They're over-estimating the likelihood of something like a terrorist attack happening, and their worrying might also mutate into worries about other things too.

Additionally, worriers can have an underlying belief that by worrying, they're increasing their protection against something bad actually happening. Perhaps they've worried about something in the past and subsequently it came true, thus confirming that it is important to think about all the possible negative outcomes. Perhaps they worry because others around them don't worry, and so they must take on the burden of worry to stop bad things happening. Unfortunately, bad things happen whether we worry about them or not (just as good things do). No one knows the future; there are multiple outcomes for every scenario, and even if they seem likely to happen, they might still not.

Worrying is not a helpful process, and is different from appraising, thinking sensibly about current risks and making decisions accordingly. That is a helpful process and you won't feel paralysed or fuelled by anxiety, and won't wake up in the middle of the night worrying. That's what we'd call problem-solving. It doesn't cause the same distress and people do not feel stuck in a worrying loop.

So worrying about what's going to happen is restrictive because no one knows what will happen. In short, the process of worry is not keeping you safe. Fortunately, worriers can benefit from the PTT approach just like anyone else suffering from an anxiety problem, and by using the same strategies. You need to work out what your beliefs about worry are, and how these beliefs are keeping the worry going, before challenging them, using the **Accept, Embrace, Control** strategy that we're describing.

Do you still need help to differentiate between getting caught up in something you can't solve and something you can solve? Then I will draw three scenarios.[18]

Scenario 1: You don't know what is going to happen in the future and therefore you can't change what eventually happens

Scenario 2: You know what's going to happen in the future and you still can't change what will happen

Scenario 3: You know what will happen in the future and you can affect the outcome of it

I'd ask in which scenario the client would place their future worry. Pretty much all worries belong in Scenarios 1 and 2. And in 100 per cent of cases, the client sees there is no point focusing on things we can't change – like the past, or things that we don't even know for certain will happen. So we can rule out Scenarios 1 and 2 as a waste of time to spend time worrying about. Only Scenario 3 is valid, because you can do something about it. However, if you can do something about it, the likelihood is you would have done this already and will not be caught up worrying about it.

For example, if you hear a rumour that your firm is making redundancies but you don't know if this is true, you can't change anything about this (Scenario 1). If they are making cuts in your department and your team, and you don't know whether it will be you or not, you still can't change this (Scenario 2), and there is no point wasting mental energy by worrying. However, if you're told that it is likely you won't have a job at Christmas, then you obviously CAN do something (Scenario 3) by looking for another job.

18 Categories of Worry strategy adopted from Dugas, M. J. & Robichaud, M. (2006), *Cognitive-Behavioral Treatment for Generalized Anxiety Disorder: From Science to Practice.* New York: Routledge; 2006.

We can break this down into another way of looking at it by introducing the **'What if?' tree**. People with anxiety problems often ask themselves 'What if?' or 'If only …' in response to threats they perceive. Adam was doing this when he bought the handcuffs to stop himself from attacking someone. He asked himself, 'What if the handcuffs aren't strong enough?' 'What if I carry the key around as well?' 'What if I throw away the key and find it again?' And so on, asking himself scores of unanswerable questions that only fuelled his anxiety. Often people blame a past event or action for their current anxiety state: 'If only I hadn't gone to the USA to train as a pilot, this problem wouldn't have happened'; 'If only I had taken that other job, then I wouldn't worry about this' and so on. People try to solve something that hasn't even happened or happened in the past because they don't want to feel the way they are feeling.

So I will draw out the 'What if?' tree, on the next page, and with reference to Adam's fear of harming others.

You'll see that as soon as you start saying, 'What if?' or 'If only' it just leads to more unanswerable questions. So the trick is to **cut off the branch** which is asking you 'What if?' or 'If only' in the first place by not answering the 'What If' question. For example, say you're having some friends round for a party and you get a knock on the door. Standing there is someone you really can't abide. Do you let them in, and ruin the evening with your friends? The 'What if?' tree might start to tell you that if you don't let the person in, you'll be thought of as rude, and you will feel guilty, etc., etc. So you let them in and, as predicted, your night is ruined and you spend the evening thinking 'If only I hadn't let them in …'

But by cutting that branch – telling the person at the door that now is not a good time – you might feel anxious for a short while because it was uncomfortable telling them they couldn't come in, but once the party is in full swing that will reduce and you will have a good time. The earlier you cut off the branch and stop trying to answer the impossible 'What if' or 'If only' questions, the quicker you will forget about them.

Another common one is **Worry about Worry** and **OCD about OCD**. I've worked with a client who has had classic OCD and thoughts

The 'What If?' Tree

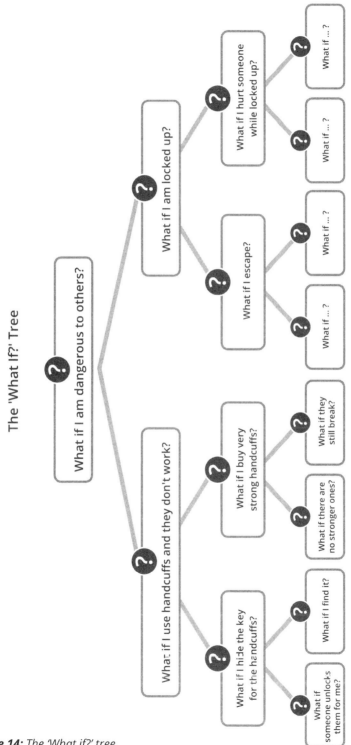

Figure 14: The 'What if?' tree.

of harming people. This has dissipated, but has been replaced by the worry that the way he experiences life and thinks about things might be wrong, and because he doesn't know whether he is right or wrong, he wonders whether all his previous intrusive thoughts and OCD might be true, and that he indeed could be a psychopath and want to harm people. The **Worry about Worry or OCD about OCD** has caused him to come full circle back to his original worry!

So that's a hard thing to challenge with exposure, and the way to deal with it is first to get him to understand that he is having an intrusive thought around worry, using the **Two Hands Theory**; in effect, his OCD is using his OCD to make him worried. So on the **One Hand**, he thinks he experiences things in life wrongly and therefore there is something wrong with him, and all his previous OCD thoughts that he is a psychopath who can never be cured must be true. On the **Other Hand**, the problem might be that he worries about the way he experiences the world, and worries that he won't have a happy future, which makes him feel very uncomfortable, and he has lost confidence in himself because of the OCD. But in essence, it is still just a worry problem so if the **Other Hand** theory is the correct one, he can now recognise the thoughts as unhelpful, and not engage with the rumination process.

We've now looked at various ways to get on top of your OCD and anxiety without resorting to your old avoidance, reassurance seeking or safety strategies. The common theme is that you've now **embraced** your OCD and anxiety, seen it for what it is and have managed to reduce your worries to a level where they're less distressing or interfering. The final part of the **PTT** approach involves the **CONTROL** of these thoughts, which we will now move on to in the next section following a summary of this one, and the conclusion from Adam.

SUMMARY

 Lauren: So let's recap what we've learned in the **Embrace** section before handing over to Adam for his thoughts about this part of the PTT approach.

We examined the idea of there being another explanation for your anxiety, to test its validity. We called this the **Two Hands Theory**. After looking at various scenarios, we found that while 'on the **One Hand**' your thoughts must be real, 'on the **Other Hand**' the problem seems to be **centred on the worry itself**, not on whether it is real.

Now we're beginning to see that the problem is one of **interpretation**, and that worry itself is not based in reality. If we accept that for what it is, we can draw it closer and by embracing it, we can diminish its power.

This is perhaps the most challenging part of our PTT approach – facing up to your fears, going towards them and allowing them to come to you. It will feel very uncomfortable at first and you might want to return to your tried-and-tested safety behaviours, compulsions and rituals. But please – have the **courage** to go towards your fears and embrace them. If you do, you will see your anxiety diminish each time you do it. This is called **habituation**.

While it feels uncomfortable and scary, the lesson is that you never know the outcome until you try.

Following this, we looked at various experiments you could do in order to embrace your anxiety and thus reduce it. By example, we showed you how to pull the trigger and by doing so, realise that your worst thoughts are just that – thoughts. We all have them, welcome or not, and by allowing them in – especially the unwelcome ones – and no longer judging them as threats, our mind will see them for what they are. And they will become less powerful.

On the next page is a table of common obsessions in OCD and experiments you can do to reduce your anxiety around them. We have also provided some examples of experiments for people with other types of anxiety problems. These are in no way exhaustive lists but hopefully you will find something you can relate to, or will help you set your own experiments:

Table 16: Suggested experiments for OCD.

Obsession	Suggested Experiments
Fear of contracting HIV from a needle	Walking past a needle exchange centre
Fear of house catching on fire from electrical fault	Leaving some lights on all day while out
Fear of being thought of as a paedophile or being a paedophile	Walking around a toy shop for twenty-five minutes or carrying a note in your wallet stating 'I am a paedophile' which you have signed
Fear of being contaminated by a specific group of people	Purposely spending time around these people
Fear of someone breaking in to your home	Leaving the door unlocked while going for a twenty-minute walk around the block
Fear of insulting God/religious deity	Writing the offensive thoughts on a piece of paper, keeping it in your pocket while attending a religious service
Fear of catching germs	Touching the door handles and taps in public toilets
Fear of throwing something away	Purposely throwing things away in a rubbish bin that is going to be collected and taken to the rubbish dump that day
Fear of not being able to stop thinking about blinking or swallowing	Purposely thinking about blinking or swallowing for thirty minutes while staring in a mirror
Fear of harming others	Standing close to other people at a busy train station or standing behind someone going down an escalator
Fear of killing yourself	Standing close to a train platform or going up a high-rise building and standing close to the edge
Fear of being sexually aroused to something unusual or unpleasant	Monitoring arousal sensations in non-trigger situations (such as just riding the bus to work or watching a game show on TV) as well as trigger situations to compare them (and see it is due to the self-focused attention and body scanning, not inappropriate thoughts)

Obsession	Suggested Experiments
Fear of being a psychopath	Purposely wishing bad things to happen to people, and see how you feel (if you feel bad or find this difficult it is very unlikely you will be a psychopath)
Fear of forgetting something important	Purposely leave something important at home that day, or don't check your bag on the way out of your home
Fear of hands not being clean enough	Purposely avoid washing hands on one day, or stop washing hands when it doesn't 'feel right'
Fear of going mad	Purposely doing things that you worry might send you mad, such as watching TV shows about mental illness
Fear that certain numbers or colours have bad things attached to them	Purposely wearing the colour and carrying around the same number of items
Fear that if things are out of order, you might never feel comfortable again, or never feel 'Just Right'	Purposely leaving things out of place for a few days such as books out of order on the bookcase and dishes by the sink, or do something else that doesn't 'feel right'
Fear of harming one's own baby or child	Changing the baby or bathing the baby without supervision or looking after the child on your own for a period of time

Table 17: Suggested experiments for other anxiety problems.

Worry	Suggested Experiments
Worry about making a mistake on an email or in a piece of work	Purposely make a small mistake in an email
Worry that people stare at you because of the way you walk	Purposely walk down the street with an exaggerated limp
Worry about a terrorist attack on a train / plane or underground train	Take a short flight, train trip or spend 30 minutes on the underground train
Fear of snakes	Visiting a pet store where they stock snakes and touching one

Worry	Suggested Experiments
Fear of making presentations or public speaking	Volunteering to do a short presentation at work, or join a debating club
Fear of driving on busy roads and motorways	Driving on a short stretch of a busy road or motorway
Worry about being late	Purposely turn up 10 minutes late
Worry about losing control of bladder in public	Drink a glass of water and take a bus ride or go to a busy place without going to the bathroom first
Fear of looking anxious at a public event (i.e. blushing or sweating)	Purposely wear warm clothes to give yourself a 'rosy' look
Fear of heights	Purposely taking the lift to the top floor of a very tall building and looking out the window
Fear of flying	Taking short flights
Worry that other people will think you are rude	Purposely do things that you think are impolite such as interrupting someone, wearing a hat inside etc.
Worry about upsetting people	Purposely saying something upsetting or not returning a phone call or email or text

In this section of the PTT approach we also looked at ways of dealing with anxiety stemming from various Thinking Problems that we've discussed previously, including **Magnified Duty**, and the role **Self-Focused Attention** and **Scanning** plays. We looked at how helpful distraction and shifting your attention can be very useful in anxiety problems. We identified a very common problem called the 'What If' tree, and that some people worry about worry, or develop OCD about OCD.

In each case, the method was rooted in the same principle – accept what it is, go towards it and embrace it, and by doing so in time your anxiety will diminish significantly.

ADAM'S CONCLUSION: EMBRACE

 Adam: As Lauren correctly points out, the most challenging part of this whole approach is embracing your OCD and anxiety for what it is. Accepting your state of mind is one thing, but actually going out and facing your fears, looking at them right in the eye and asking them to come to you – well, that takes real courage. If this is where you are at the moment, you have my respect and admiration as I have been in that exact place. The hardest thing is welcoming this stuff in; the very things that have been giving you nightmares for years and have ruined your life are now on the doorstep, and you're expected to open the door and let them into the party. That's not easy, and it takes courage in spades.

During the period when I was accepting my state of mind, I did go through a blip and had a bad period of OCD where I became very aware of my sensory functions; swallowing and blinking, as we have mentioned. I quickly became very anxious about these natural sensory behaviours in that I would always be conscious of them and therefore would never be able to take my mind off them. It became quite distressing as I had fallen back into the trap (without me even realising) of trying to get rid of these thoughts. I started putting a lot of effort into trying not to think about it (creating a safety behaviour, of course), which as we know is completely the wrong thing to do. However, Lauren immediately spotted this and put me right back on track. My OCD and anxiety had just simply latched onto something else.

Instead of running away and trying to distract myself, I went straight to the OCD around my sensory functions and instead thought about them as much as I could. Lauren also kept on reminding me non-stop, to the point where she'd remind me at random times via text message, even late in the evening. That felt very difficult and I'd think, 'You must be kidding – now you'll set me off!' Which was exactly the point. To get a grip of OCD and anxiety you need to embrace it as tightly as this. Lauren taught me to make time to bring on my anxieties, to deliberately think about blinking and swallowing.

Eventually I learned to allow my thoughts in, to do the worst they could to me, by lying down for ten minutes and thinking, 'Come on in, you're welcome to ten minutes of my mind. Just do what you want.' I'd lie there and let every thought pass through me. By doing so, I accepted and embraced them, seeing them for what they were – just thoughts and an arousal of fear, but without any substance behind it.

As you'll remember, when I first met Lauren I was suffering from severe panic attacks, and even the thought of them was enough to bring one on. I had them so many times a day I'd lose count, and would go to bed completely exhausted. Lauren helped me to accept that I might get them, which was fine, but she told me that I needed to embrace them to make them stop. One day, she suggested we go for a drive and once we'd parked up, she asked me to try to bring on a panic attack. She sat there and started to say things which would deliberately raise my anxiety levels; she told me that I would have anxiety for the rest of my life, that I would never get better, and what was I going to do about that? She presented me with all the triggers that would normally induce a panic attack within seconds. And yet, when I pulled that trigger and tried to bring on an attack, I just couldn't do it – proving that what I feared most was the **worry** that I'd have an attack. When I tried to make myself have one, it didn't happen. There was no substance behind it at all. It just didn't have the fuel necessary to proceed to the stages of a full-blown panic attack. I had cut off its source of fuel; the fear. I did this by facing the fear and embracing it.

To me, that proved just how powerful the concept of **Embrace** is. You can run forever, or fight like hell, but you'll never win. But in a complete turnaround of whatever you've previously thought, by embracing your anxiety you will see it for what it is and overcome it, because your mind is desensitised to it. That knowledge helped me to see the bigger picture, which is that anxiety is based on fear, and it's false. Eventually I was able to pick up a knife in Lauren's presence and put it to her neck as well as to my own. I felt no fear, because I knew I had no aspiration to stab anyone. In fact, I couldn't think of anything I wanted to do less! I accepted my previous thought – that I was going to harm someone – as just a thought, and now I knew it was based on the worry about that thought. By embracing that thought, testing it out with the knife, I knew it was 100 per cent false.

I'm aware that people have multiple OCD issues and anxieties around many different things, and that they treat each one as a separate 'fight'. Under the PTT approach there is simply no need. Eventually, your mind will recognise that OCD and anxiety is nothing but a lie. It's a false rumour, which likes to hype itself up and sound convincing, but in reality it has nothing; all it has is the power you actually give it, and by embracing the thought, you give it no power. Over a period of time you won't even need to think about the process of challenging it any more. Your mind will do the work for you by naturally filtering away the intrusive thoughts and leaving the ones that are relevant and useful for day-to-day living.

It's important that you've carefully read our PTT approach so far, as described by Lauren. I know there is a lot to take in, and you may be resistant at first. That is fine, and it's perfectly normal. The PTT approach is probably contrary to everything you've believed, and it will certainly be counter to anything you've done in terms of 'fighting' your anxiety and OCD. Remember, we are not 'fighting', we are using courage. Essentially, we're asking you to adopt a simple philosophy, which is to **ACCEPT** your anxiety for what it is and **EMBRACE** it so that you become desensitised to it. The final element in our approach is understanding how to **CONTROL** it. Again, this is very different from what you might expect!

SECTION 3

CONTROL

Lauren: You are now at a point where you can start to see how your anxiety is able to reduce noticeably. Hopefully you may have already started to implement the PTT approach into your life and are now starting to witness the results first hand. You've followed the **Accept** and **Embrace** strategies we've shown you and you're discovering they will work for you. Now you stand on the threshold of a life free from anxiety and related depression. But for how long will you feel this way? What happens if those intrusive and unwelcome thoughts come tumbling back into your mind? Are you strong enough to deal with them or will you be blindsided by thoughts you imagined you'd never encounter again?

To answer these questions, we need to look at how you will take **CONTROL** during your period of recovery. Perhaps the most important point to make in this section, from the outset, is that **Control** is not about control at all, at least not in the usual sense of the word. This isn't about controlling your anxiety or OCD by finding ways of keeping it at bay – as we know, you've been doing that for years using ritual and safety responses, and it hasn't worked and you now know it will never work.

The way to control your OCD and anxiety is to allow it in. Let it come to you, or go to it, and ask it to sit with you.

It sounds counter-intuitive, doesn't it? 'After all this time,' you might ask, 'you're telling me not to ignore my anxiety, but to make friends with it?'

Well, in a way, yes. You don't want to feel a certain way, whether it be anxious, depressed, frustrated, sad and so on. These are strong emotions, even if they are normal ones experienced by all of us at one time or another, to different degrees of intensity. All emotions can escalate and feel very uncomfortable, but in time they reduce naturally and more so if we are accepting of them.

The problem is that, as a society, we are sometimes taught that feeling uncomfortable is wrong, and that if we have even a twinge of an unpleasant emotion we need to solve it immediately. If you're depressed you need to be happy, so take a pill. If your relationship isn't right you need to fix it right away. We're taught that life should be perfect and if it isn't, you must do something about it.

To my mind, that doesn't fit with us being human. It is normal to feel strong emotions, even if they are uncomfortable. When someone dies we grieve, but we don't grieve in the same way forever. Eventually grief reduces and while life might never be the same again without that person, it goes on. It has to. Accepting and embracing the fact that we all have strong emotions – that we can all feel anxious, worried, scared, depressed, etc. – is the key to recovering from OCD and anxiety, and maintaining that recovery for the rest of your life.

As we've said, when people feel strong emotions, they very often do something to try and get rid of those feelings. Sometimes it works and they stop feeling anxious straight away. But as we know, the person then moves into the vicious cycle of anxiety, which feeds on their anxiety; making it worse and requiring more and more rituals and safety behaviours to make the feelings go away. Unfortunately, the feelings never actually go away – they are just hidden for a short time and will always re-emerge because you haven't dealt with your anxiety – you are just avoiding it with rituals, and safety behaviours. What we know from **Accept** and **Embrace** is that if we allow those feelings in, they will reduce. And when the feelings reduce, that is the time to challenge the thinking which lies beneath the emotion.

On the next page is a graph showing what I like to call the '**Impermanence of emotions**'. You will see that your anxiety level will rise but if you sit with it, accepting it for what it is and embracing it, the level of intensity will eventually drop. All emotions, regardless of how intense or frequent, will eventually reduce. If you think about how you were feeling when you got up this morning, or when you first picked up this book, or when you had lunch, you will note that your feelings will be **different**, either in the feeling you experience or in its intensity. This means that both unpleasant and pleasant feelings will not last forever, even if you think they will! In the midst of severe anxiety or depression, it is hard to believe this but ...

ALL FEELINGS EVENTUALLY CHANGE AND ALL STRONG FEELINGS EVENTUALLY REDUCE.

It is a fact.

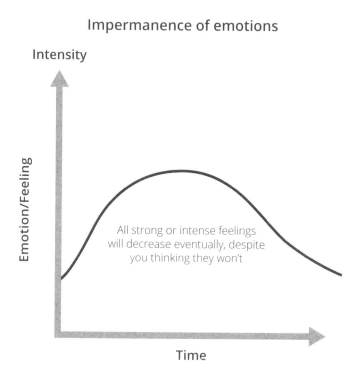

Figure 15: Impermanence of emotions.

Most people worry that strong, unpleasant feelings will last forever or even continue to get worse, and try to stop feeling that way by using a safety response to avoid it or reduce it. However, if you employ a tried-and-tested safety response, as you've always done, you might experience some drop, but in actuality over time you're maintaining that anxiety.

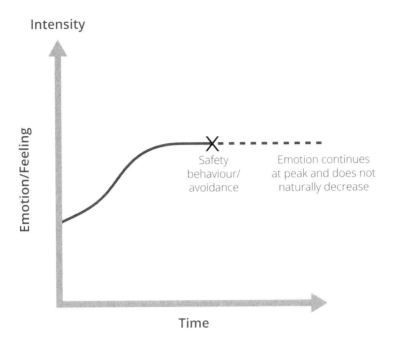

Figure 16: *Effect of safety behaviour or avoidance on our emotions.*

If you have experienced a course of CBT or even used some of the strategies in this book to challenge your thinking, you may try to use these straight away when you feel intensely anxious – and with dismay find that they don't seem to work. 'Hold on,' you think, 'I'm following what the therapist said/the strategies in this book but it's not working – I'm still feeling anxious!' This is because your body is also in fight, flight or freeze mode (we talked about this earlier) and it will naturally feel in an anxious state because of the build-up of the stress hormones adrenalin, norepinephrine and cortisol. Once activated, this fight, flight or freeze process can take up to thirty minutes for the hormones to leave the body. This makes it much harder to be logical and reason dispassionately when our body is telling us 'high alert – there is a threat'. So it's not that your strategies to challenge your thinking are not working or won't work; your body is still in threat mode so it is too hard to 'believe' them at that point. What I suggest is to 'get through' the feeling, and once your emotion is less intense and your body has had a chance to calm down physiologically, then you can practise your thought-challenging.

So instead of avoiding the feeling, allow it in and sit with it. And **take a compassionate response** to it.

What do we mean by this? It means accepting that you feel this way, not judging yourself for it and understanding that no matter how intense, the emotion is not permanent. If you accept this, then you can choose to do something different in that moment. Not by way of avoiding the feeling, but by a compassionate diversion which acknowledges that while you feel bad now, you won't feel so bad forever. So this could constitute something simple like going for a walk or a jog, reading a book, listening to music or making a meal or baking. You're not trying to stop or avoid the feeling. You're just being kind to yourself. I call this **helpful distraction** – acknowledging the feeling but choosing to do something distracting to be kind to yourself, and allowing the feeling to naturally reduce in intensity.

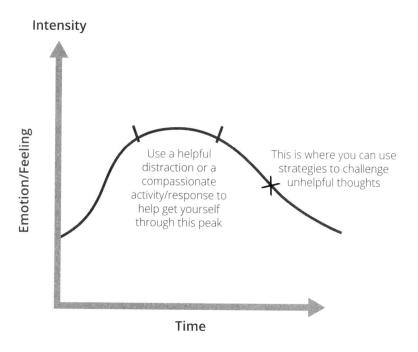

Figure 17: *How to manage strong emotions / feelings.*

I had a person in therapy for his OCD who felt he couldn't function while he was feeling intensely anxious. He had problems paying his bills, checking his online banking situation, using the phone, tidying up – basically, anything household-related. His fear was that his state of mind would prevent him from doing these properly, and that if he did them while anxious it would be a disaster. By seeing that he didn't have to feel 100 per cent OK to carry out a few household tasks, I was able to help him see that he didn't have to pay any special attention to the tasks – he just carried them out when he was feeling anxious, and he changed the meaning he attached to the feeling (that it was intolerable and meant that he couldn't do anything properly) to 'it is OK not to feel OK and I can still get on with my life despite this feeling'.

So we are treating the feeling by not avoiding it, but we're doing it in a compassionate way for ourselves. **It is OK not to feel OK, because you are a human, and that is part of being human.**

As time moves on and you understand that you must accept and embrace your anxiety, and that controlling it means not controlling it, but looking after yourself with compassion, you will notice your anxiety lessening. Progress is being made, your mood is lifted and you feel that a much brighter future is ahead.

Ironically, it's at this point where people can really go to pieces if they have a bad day. You're feeling generally better and you are noticing progress, so a bad day can really provoke a lot of agonising and 'this hasn't worked for me!' or 'there's no point now as treatment clearly hasn't worked'. This is normal. Recovering from an anxiety-based, or obsessional, illness is like recovering from any illness in that there will be ups and downs before a complete recovery is made. If you imagine you're a regular runner and you're recovering from tendonitis (an inflamed tendon), there will be days when you want to, and are able to, gently jog round the park or along the riverbank, but there will be days when it is too painful and you can't run as far as you would like to. The fact is that you have to be compassionate to yourself and give time for the injury to heal properly before you can do this. Those can be days filled with frustration, irritation and despair that you will never complete your goal of running long distances again.

Just as tendonitis doesn't last forever, neither does a spell of anxiety.

If you're feeling down about having had a bad day, allow yourself that feeling, because it is normal. The problems arise when you attach a meaning to the feeling and there is a thinking problem in that meaning, usually **catastrophising**, such as 'I am not getting better', 'I will never get better', 'This is a waste of time'. If you didn't have up and down days you wouldn't be making progress, and I would be more concerned about that than a few 'off-days' among the better ones.

Have a look at the **Recovery Graph** below and this is what we would expect in recovering from an anxiety or obsessional problem. The general trend is in the right direction, but there will be peaks and troughs along the journey:

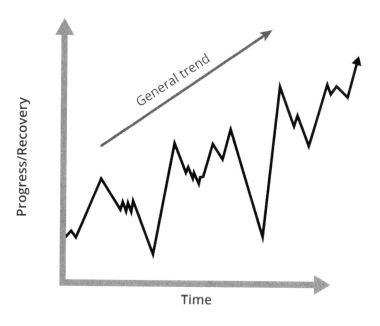

Figure 18: *Progress and recovery over time.*

As we've mentioned before, you can get OCD about OCD (and anxiety about anxiety), and the most common time for this is during the recovery phase. You are on the road to a brighter future and the last thing you want now is to have another episode of anxiety or OCD because this threatens your recovery. You've had such a traumatic time that you worry the clock will be turned back to the bad old days when your OCD and anxiety had you in a powerful grip.

So the threat of this happening becomes the worry itself, and people who experience anxiety about anxiety and OCD about OCD will start body-scanning, checking their responses and avoiding situations that might make them anxious – in short, going back to the tried-and-tested methods which haven't worked and in fact made things worse. As we've said, there are two ways of seeing this; **on the One Hand**, your OCD or anxiety problem is going to return and you will be back in that desperate place trapped by anxiety, or **on the Other Hand**, you are **worried** that your OCD or anxiety problem will come back as it was such a difficult time for you, but the problem is that you are **worried** about it (rather than it actually happening). Which theory best fits your experience? If it's the latter, then accept and embrace these fears, and by seeing them for what they are you will learn to control them.

A little later in the book we will hear about Adam's OCD and anxiety from his wife Alissa's perspective, but at this point I would like to say something about family involvement in this type of anxiety disorder as it does have some bearing on recovery.

We can all agree that it's awful to see a family member in distress, and when this happens the natural human instinct is to reach out to help or reassure them. That's normal behaviour and it's a highly effective solution when it applies to many different illnesses, especially physical ones. But as we know, reassurance is a friend of anxiety and far from curing it, actually makes it worse. If we reassure our family member or friend suffering from OCD or an anxiety problem, we help to turn the vicious cycle even faster.

And yet, we don't like to see those close to us suffer. So if you're reading this book and PTT approach because you want to understand and help a friend or relative with OCD or an anxiety problem, or you're a sufferer and need help in a constructive way, then please read on.

We need to help those suffering from OCD and anxiety-related disorders in a caring, compassionate but non-reassuring way, and this is a fine line to walk. For example, if your relative or friend has OCD around fear of contamination, he or she may seek reassurance that the shopping you brought home was only touched by people with clean hands, that you washed your hands immediately after handling cash, and that you will now wash all the fruit and vegetables before they are eaten. The obvious response is to say, 'Yes, don't worry, I did all those things ...'

That, however, feeds the OCD by reassuring it. What you need to say is, 'I know you're worried and I understand that, but I'm not giving in to your OCD so I won't reassure you that I've done these things ...'

OK, that might sound a little harsh, but if it is done in a caring and compassionate way it is the right approach to take. Reassurance might feel better, but it won't help. On the contrary, it could make things worse for the whole family. I had a client who was so worried about contamination that she insisted that her husband strip off his clothes on the back porch before he entered the house on coming home from work, and then shower in a separate bathroom. As you'd imagine, this was difficult and uncomfortable for him, especially in winter. But he did it because he loved his wife and didn't want to see her suffer, yet it was interfering in his life as well as hers.

So family members can unwittingly collude in OCD and anxiety, and if this is you, you need to ask yourself, 'Am I doing anything to feed into this, allowing it to grow?' If so, that is the point at which you intervene by stopping complying with your relative or friend's requests. It might mean that the sufferer becomes frustrated and annoyed. They might even say, 'You don't love me any more, because if you did you would reassure me that everything is OK.' But you need to have the conversation with the sufferer that ends in the agreement that you will not reassure and feed into their anxiety, no matter how uncomfortable this might feel. A whole family can suffer through OCD or an anxiety problem because it is restricting their lives, but they need to be healthy in order to care for the sufferer who isn't feeling those things.

Just because you're not reassuring doesn't mean you're selfish. You can be supportive without colluding. If you recall the experiments we looked at in the last section, you'll remember that I said that those undertaking them can be supported by a friend or family member **so long as that doesn't become a safety behaviour**. If they're worried they might hit someone while driving, and that fear is restricting their mobility, then go out with them in the car and just sit with them without reassuring them. Then let them go out on their own, and when they arrive home ask them how it went. Both the sufferer and their family or friends can agree upon a system of support which doesn't rely upon reassurance, and in the 'Family' section later in this book Alissa will describe how she worked with Adam to achieve this.

Nonetheless, I acknowledge that it can be very difficult for families to see loved ones in distress, particularly when it involves young people. Parents can become incredibly distressed and will protect their children from the downsides of OCD or anxiety-based illnesses – thereby keeping the problem going. It can also go the other way, in that the parent or caregiver with OCD or anxiety problems, worries that their anxiety is so consuming that they are unable to connect emotionally with their children and will therefore damage their development. Although we are not in the business of reassurance, what we can say is that many people experience mental health problems in life, including parents and caregivers. Think about the message you are sending your children from accepting and embracing the anxiety problem and getting better – that even though things were really difficult, you had the strength to change things and get yourself into better mental health. That is the role model that children need and the message they can take forward in life. In a way, OCD and anxiety can be seen as akin to an addiction problem, in that the sufferer may have to get worse, and be in difficult, uncomfortable situations, in order to get better. That can be hard for other people to comprehend but it's often what is needed for recovery.

To sum up, once you've learned about OCD and anxiety, you've looked at interventions, done the experiments, challenged your safety behaviours and learned to recognise the signs of OCD and anxiety, it's time to take what I call a 'helicopter view' of your anxiety disorder. This is when you no longer have to go into the detail and the content of everything we've discussed and learned – you merely sit back and observe the process without noticing too much about its detail. It's a bit like a train journey; if it's new to you, you're noticing everything around you – the colour of the seats, the adverts, the destinations, the scenery going by, the stations you arrive at. You are probably paying attention to every stop just in case it is the one you need, and you analyse every announcement made by the conductor in case it affects your travel. However, if you take this journey time after time, such things become familiar to you. You know where you need to be and you simply follow the process of taking the train journey. You will stop paying attention to every stop or announcement that is made. And you will trust yourself to pay attention when you need to rather than being hyper-vigilant the whole journey, paying attention to every detail. When you reach this stage with OCD and anxiety you are stepping above the theory; you don't need to work out what it is, so you go straight to the process without becoming embedded in the content. You don't need to work out where it fits in the 'on the **One Hand**, or on the **Other Hand**'. You will just know it is a worry problem and you need to manage your feelings, and get through the situation rather than challenge the thoughts. This doesn't mean you won't need to do some embracing and exposure – even with the exposures you will just know when you need to do one rather than analysing it in detail.

For example, if Adam has intrusive thoughts about harming people, because he understands and accepts his OCD he no longer needs to challenge the interpretation (**on the One Hand** vs. **on the Other Hand**) or do experiments to embrace it. He knows that it is an intrusion and the anxiety is a feeling, and he doesn't have to do anything about it. He can choose to just leave the thoughts where they are (accept), feel a little uncomfortable (embrace), but get on with his life. This is recognising the process of the OCD or anxiety problem and not needing to go into the details.

SUMMARY

Lauren: So let's now summarise briefly what we learned in **CONTROL**, then hand over to Adam for the conclusion.

The main point to make about '**Control**' is that it is not about control at all, at least not in the conventional sense. If you're trying to control something, it usually means you're having a battle with it and that's the opposite of what we need to do to recover from anxiety.

What we're asking you to do is control your anxiety by allowing it in.

Accepting and embracing your anxiety and OCD, seeing it for what it is, is the key to controlling it. You aren't letting it 'win' – you're simply accepting what it is, and going forward to meet your anxiety head-on. Every time you do this you are in control, because you will find that with every embrace the level of your anxiety drops downwards, while the rate of your recovery heads upwards.

However, you will have 'bad' days as well as good ones. This is perfectly normal. Don't avoid those bad days; allow them in, sit with them and treat yourself with compassion. This means being kind to yourself while anxiety is upon you, and getting on with your life by doing the things you normally do. This isn't avoiding or running away or carrying out a safety behaviour; it's what I would describe as 'helpful distraction'.

Remember – it's OK not to feel OK.

Part of the **CONTROL** aspect of your recovery might involve your family and friends. Take time to explain the PTT approach to them and do not let them reassure you about your anxiety problem or OCD – as we know, that will form part of a safety behaviour. Make an agreement that they will support you in a compassionate way, and that you will not make any demands for reassurance. It's a fine line to walk, but a worthwhile one.

Finally, when you feel your feeling of anxiety has dropped to a level you're comfortable with, and appears to be staying that way, you can go to a 'helicopter view' of it. This is when you no longer need to recall everything we've learned and work through the detail because your mind has now understood the cycle of anxiety and its patterns, and is now able to step above it, notice it and choose when to intervene if necessary.

ADAM'S CONCLUSION: CONTROL

 Adam: When I first met Lauren I was very poorly indeed, and when I look back now I see how from childhood I was plagued with extreme anxiety. I never knew what it was like to be normal and to have a normal mindset. So the realisation that, for the first time in my life, I was getting better was an incredibly powerful and moving one. It's the image of myself as an anxious little boy which now motivates me to continue my recovery every single day of my life and, through The Shaw Mind Foundation (www.shawmindfoundation.org), to help others who are suffering as I did.

That realisation came about when I first started to feel more control over my illness. I began to see that I was allowing myself to sit with my thoughts and not beat myself up about them. It dawned on me that to be in control, it was fine NOT to be in control. A contradiction in terms, I know, but one that works perfectly. I realised that it was OK to accept any thoughts coming into my head, and that it was alright for me to be fearful of confronting (or embracing) my fears. Trying to control your thoughts is like trying to flatten water: the more you try to flatten the water, the more waves you make. When I understood that, I also understood that I had at last got my sanity back.

Now I knew that my OCD and anxiety had been controlling me, all my life. And that's because I fought and questioned, questioned and fought. In short, I'd been feeding a monster that eventually controlled and nearly destroyed me. I didn't see that I was fearful of fear, anxious about becoming anxious. It took the strategy of **Accept**, **Embrace** and **Control** for me to gain clarity, understand and work this out.

For me, to be 'in control' means going towards my anxiety, embracing it, sitting with it – even welcoming it in. I control my sanity by understanding that I can't and don't control my thoughts and emotions. If anxiety comes on, I go to it. And when I do, the unwanted thought is nowhere near as bad as it once was. In fact, it's died off, and that's because I've desensitised myself to it and the brain has simply stopped developing unwanted and intrusive thoughts, or in reality is no longer in tune to them if such a thought occurs. They are now nothing more than a minor inconvenience so my mind naturally filters them away. I can go a couple of weeks without them now and in a strange way that can be disappointing, because I like the opportunity to welcome them in, to see them for what they are. Every time this happens, I feel stronger. Regarding OCD and anxiety, I don't ever think, 'I've beaten you' because that puts it in the context of a fight. My attitude is that it is, and always will be, a part of me, and I need to learn to live with that. What I will not do is allow it to control me.

In short, anxiety is what it is. Thoughts are just thoughts, nothing else. And we need these thoughts as humans, to learn, live and evolve. A meaning can attach itself to a thought – so accept it and let it be there. If it causes us further anxiety, move towards it, embrace it, and then you'll see how much power it has. Consequently this may cause us to experience strong unpleasant emotions. Again accepting, and allowing yourself to feel these is key. It only has power and growth if you give it that, by fighting it. But if you face and embrace your fear and accept that sometimes you'll feel bad, you will see how quickly its power shrinks.

That, in a nutshell, is what Pulling the Trigger is all about.

SECTION 4

DEPRESSION AND PANIC ATTACKS – THE BY-PRODUCTS OF ANXIETY

 Lauren: In the course of this book and PTT approach we've mentioned both depression and panic attacks. Adam suffered from both and it's not surprising, given that both are very common by-products of OCD and anxiety.

Consider this for a moment: anxiety has stripped you of the life you were living, a life free of worry and torment. You can barely function without feeling anxious, and the only way to set aside the feelings is to repeat rituals or safety behaviours over and over again. Your mind is constantly invaded by unpleasant thoughts, to the point where you wonder what is normal and what isn't.

In those circumstances, it's hardly surprising that many, if not most, OCD and anxiety sufferers also experience depression and panic attacks. In my practice I rarely meet sufferers who haven't had one or both. However, I would also say that while both depression and panic attacks are deeply uncomfortable, they are **normal** experiences and there are things you can do to alleviate them without having to adopt avoidance techniques or safety behaviours. I've outlined some of these below, and at the end of each section Adam has applied his conclusion directly from the sufferer's point of view, commenting on his feelings towards panic attacks and depression, and how he dealt with both in order to now live a life free from panic attacks and depression.

DEPRESSION

As I've said, it's perfectly normal to experience clinical depression as a result of OCD and anxiety. The latter has reduced your functioning capability, affected your relationships and prevented you from enjoying the things you used to. More than 40 per cent of people with OCD and anxiety have what we call 'co-morbid' depression; diagnosable clinical depression occurring alongside OCD and anxiety.

At this stage, I think it's useful to point out again that we are discussing **depression as a result of OCD and anxiety**. Depression that was around before OCD and anxiety may need separate treatment not covered in the confines of this book. If this is the case, you do need to see your medical practitioner for further advice. For further information and help on depression please visit www.shawmindfoundation.org.

We would define **Major Depressive Disorder** as having low mood for more than two weeks, plus **five** of the following symptoms[19]:

- feeling tearful and hopeless
- reduced interest in pleasurable activities
- significant weight gain or loss
- insomnia or hypersomnia (sleeping too much or too little)
- sluggishness
- feeling tired
- loss of energy
- feeling worthless or excessively guilty
- not being able to think
- inability to concentrate or make decisions
- thoughts of suicide.

While we may all experience some of these symptoms from time to time, the key is if you have had low mood consistently for the past two weeks and at least five of the other symptoms, then you are probably depressed. Some people find the 'thoughts of suicide' worrying and frightening. You may think that you don't deserve to be around any more, that people would be better off with you not around, or that you simply can't deal with life any longer. While many

19 American Psychiatric Association. (2013). *Diagnostic and Statistical Manual of Mental Disorders* (5th ed.). Arlington, VA: American Psychiatric Publishing.

people with depression have these types of thoughts, as a clinician I would be very concerned if you wanted to kill yourself and found comfort in these thoughts, or had made a plan to kill yourself, or had tried to kill yourself in the past. If that were the case I would ask you to seek direct professional help immediately. For further information, please visit www.shawmindfoundation.org.

However, and slightly confusingly, we are not talking about intrusive thoughts about suicide as part of OCD. I have worked with a number of people who have had intrusive thoughts about committing suicide, and therefore worry that they want to kill themselves and are at risk of doing so. The difference in this situation is that the intrusive thoughts cause intense anxiety and lead to the person avoiding any situations in which they worry they might be able to cause themselves harm. In contrast, in depression, thoughts of suicide do not lead to this extensive avoidance or reassurance seeking, and often the thoughts don't cause such anxiety found in OCD.

There are other types of depression people can get alongside an anxiety problem. One familiar to OCD and anxiety sufferers is **Persistent Depressive Disorder (PDD)**[20] (previously known as **Dysthymic Disorder)**, which is a persistent but slightly less severe low mood. If you have Persistent Depressive Disorder your mood will have been low for most of the day, more days than not, for at least two years. Alongside the low mood you will have **two** of the following symptoms: low appetite, low energy, low self-esteem, poor concentration, feelings of hopelessness and difficulty making decisions. You haven't had a reprieve from these symptoms for longer than two months in those two years. Persistent Depressive Disorder may not have the same symptom severity at once as Major Depressive Disorder, but is chronic and constant.

Both these depressive disorders are debilitating, and can actually affect the process of recovery from OCD and anxiety. If you're feeling down, you're not sleeping or eating properly and your motivation is barely existent, you're unlikely to be up and ready for the challenge of freeing yourself from OCD and anxiety. The good news is that if you do try the treatment strategies outlined in the PTT approach, it's

---

20 American Psychiatric Association. (2013). *Diagnostic and Statistical Manual of Mental Disorders* (5th ed.). Arlington, VA: American Psychiatric Publishing.

more than likely you will find the depression lifting gradually. But to start that process we need to address the issue of depression first.

Firstly, and indeed from a professional view, I would consider whether the sufferer might benefit from medication. We will go into this subject in more detail later in the PTT approach. Suffice to say that a lot of medication used to treat anxiety by medical specialists is also prescribed for depression, and if you're co-morbidly depressed it might be useful to speak with a medical specialist to consider medication. This could provide the boost you need as a sufferer of depression and anxiety; the step that allows you to start getting better.

However, if you take medication you will still need to follow the methods that challenge your thinking and behaviour, as outlined in the PTT approach.

Medication can be a useful starting point if you're anxious and depressed, but it is by no means a cure-all. Research suggests it can be a useful way of kick-starting your recovery, and if someone had chronic diabetes or a physical injury we wouldn't question that medication has its place. That said, not everyone with depression needs medication, so let's look at some other strategies to help ourselves make progress and get better.

Sleep is one of the major keys in recovery from depression, along with **eating** and **exercise**. Anxiety, OCD and depression can throw out sleep patterns to such an extent that sufferers find their day turns into night, and vice versa. If this unstable pattern persists, it's hardly surprising that it can affect a person's mood very strongly. Think how you are if you miss a night's sleep, then multiply this by seven nights on the trot and you begin to get the idea of how poor sleep intrudes into your mental well-being. I've talked to people who can't sleep and spend most of their evenings doing their OCD rituals and trying to make things OK. Then they wake up in the afternoon and wonder why they feel so terrible. It is also very common for anxiety sufferers to lie awake plagued by their worries, so they don't ever feel refreshed in the morning.

If you are lying in bed worrying about things, one thing to try is either distract yourself with a good book or listen to some soothing music, and practice shifting your attention as we have discussed earlier in the book. Or, and I appreciate this is very hard, try and delay your worries like the OCD sufferer delaying their rituals. You can always come back to them in the morning and worry about them then. The worries are unlikely to change over the course of a night. Some people find it helpful to write down their worries on a notepad beside the bed, so they remember to worry about them in the morning. Although what we usually find is that the worries don't seem as important or urgent in the morning as they were the previous night!

If you're still at the stage where you are up very late because you're completing rituals, let me suggest that you begin these earlier so that you can get to bed at a more reasonable hour. Better still, if you can, delay them until the following morning. I know this is contrary to other advice in the PTT approach, but in this particular case you absolutely need sleep and energy to help your recovery.

Your sleep is very important and you need to get back into a solid sleeping pattern.

This doesn't mean that you should go to bed at 9pm and sleep until 8am the following day. Around six to eight hours' sleep is enough for anyone. What matters is that you get into a regular pattern of sleep by going to bed at the same time each night – 11pm or midnight, say – and getting up at the same time the following morning, for example, 6am or 7am. Initially this may be hard to do but if you stick to it you will find that in a week or so you are in a regular pattern. If possible, avoid alcohol, caffeine or any other stimulants before you go to bed. You might assume that a few glasses of wine will knock you out, but the quality of sleep you get will be poor. Also, cut out any naps you may be having in the day. You may feel tired in the afternoon – many of us do after lunch – but refrain from napping. This can also interfere with your natural sleep rhythm and make it harder to sleep at night or develop regular patterns.

You might find that you're going to bed at the correct time but you still can't sleep. This can be annoying, and it can also provoke anxiety in that you start worrying about why you're not sleeping. If you haven't dropped off in twenty-five to thirty minutes, don't lie in bed fighting feelings of frustration; get up and do something else until your body feels tired. Perhaps read a book or have a bath or a shower, complete a crossword or sip a herbal tea. Try not to do anything too stimulating as you will find it hard to go back to bed. Once you start to feel tired, go back to bed and try again. You may have to repeat this, but there is no point lying in bed not sleeping and getting anxious about it – it will become an unpleasant experience, and being anxious will make it even harder to get to sleep, and sleep should be a relaxing time. As ever, treat yourself with compassion and don't be hard on yourself, and accept your thoughts, emotions and sensations.

Adam will mention his approach to diet and exercise in Section 5, and how paying attention to both really helped him with his recovery. His practical advice is very useful and well worth following. With depression, we either experience loss of appetite or we gain weight because we're eating 'comfort foods' that aren't good for our bodies. The body needs good quality fuel to perform its tasks, and if you're experiencing depression it is useful to look at your diet to see if you can make changes. Eat regularly, and substitute foods high in fat, sugar and salt with more healthy options. Introducing a period of exercise each day can result in a huge boost in your motivation, releasing lots of important endorphins and helping you sleep better at night. As Adam will demonstrate in Section 5, finding the motivation to begin regular exercise when you're depressed can be hard at first, but if you build it up from short periods (five to ten minutes is fine) you will notice significant improvement in your mood.

If you have depression, you'll more than likely notice that you've stopped doing the things you used to enjoy. Where you used to swim regularly or meet up with friends after work, you now find excuses to go home and sit in front of the TV. Even the thought of catching the bus to the pool or chatting to colleagues in the bar makes you feel exhausted. Depression depletes energy, the enjoyment and sense of achievement we get from things, and in turn this starts a 'vicious cycle' – very similar to the model we examined for anxiety – of not putting any effort in and therefore getting nothing back. To remedy this, we need a **Behaviour Booster**.[21]

21 Dimidjian, S., Hollon, S. D., Dobson, K. S., Schmaling, K. B., Kohlenberg, R. J., Addis, M. E., and Atkins, D. C. (2006). Randomized trial of behavioral activation, cognitive therapy, and antidepressant medication in the acute treatment of adults with major depression. *Journal of Consulting and Clinical Psychology*, 74(4), 658.

Using a scale, let's look at an activity you enjoyed before depression set in. As an example, I'll use swimming:

BEFORE DEPRESSION

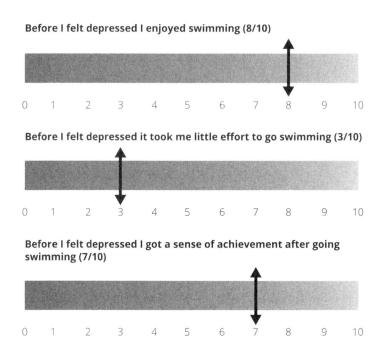

Figure 19: Enjoyment, effort and sense of achievement before depression.

You'll see that you might score 8/10 on the Enjoyment scale, and 7/10 on the Achievement scale, whereas it took little effort (3/10) to motivate yourself to go swimming.

Now let's look at the same scale during the onset of depression, and figure out how you felt when you last went swimming.

DURING A DEPRESSED EPISODE

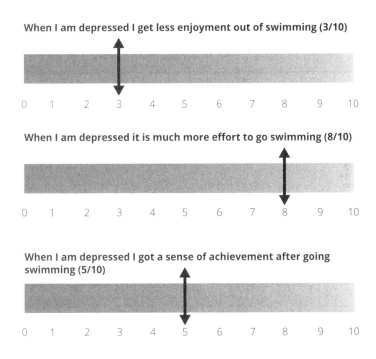

Figure 20: *Enjoyment, effort and sense of achievement during a depressed episode.*

Now you'll see some of the scales are exactly the opposite; that you get little enjoyment from swimming, feel that you have achieved less as you have only swum half the distance you normally do, and have to make a much bigger effort to actually get to the pool. Hence why people stop doing the things they enjoy as it takes so much more effort to get such little enjoyment or they feel less effective; it hardly seems worth it to them.

So if we examine the situation now, in the middle of depression, let's see what happens when you simply avoid going swimming:

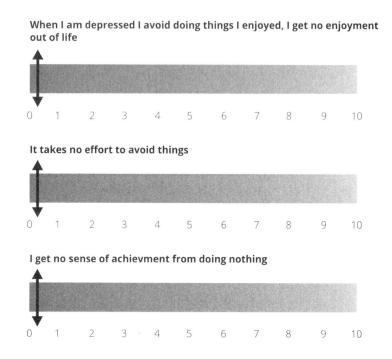

Figure 21: *Effect of avoidance on enjoyment, effort and sense of achievement.*

The depression has you in such a strong grip that you are not getting any enjoyment or much of a sense of achievement from swimming or any other activity, so you avoid it, as you are not getting any enjoyment or feeling effective at all! But look again at Figure 20. Are you able to extract that little bit of enjoyment, despite the effort you have to make, to go swimming? If you at least make the effort, you are highly likely to find that it wasn't as bad as you thought, and that you maybe even got more than 3/10 along the enjoyment scale. This is much better than 0/10 on the scale. Similarly, you will still get a sense of achievement from going swimming, even if you swim half the distance you used to.

This is the **Behaviour Booster**, and using this scale is an excellent way of persuading those suffering from OCD, anxiety and related depression to see that while they might only experience a small amount of enjoyment or get less of a sense of achievement from an activity compared to what they used to, it is better than not having any enjoyment at all and feeling ineffectual. From this we can then devise a diary in which the sufferer plans a few activities ahead; nothing too heavy or too taxing, but small things which help us reconnect with the pleasures we once enjoyed, or to feel effective again. There may be obstacles ahead, but note those down too and work out a way of getting around them in advance. Setting achievable goals is an excellent way of achieving the **Behaviour Booster**, which in turn will help to lift the depression and get you motivated to deal with your OCD and anxiety.

To help, fill in the box below. You should select activities that you used to enjoy, or ones that gave you a sense of being effective or achieving something:

Table 18: Design your own behaviour booster.

My activities this week are ...

I plan to do these activities on the following days at the following time (e.g. Wednesday afternoon)

After the activity describe how it went below. How much effort did it take? How much enjoyment did you get from it? Did you get a sense of achievement?

What obstacles did you overcome in order to complete this activity?

Mark your rating from 1 to 10

Enjoyment [   ]   Effort [   ]   Achievement [   ]

Another way of examining depression in the context of OCD and anxiety is to look at **Thinking Problems**. We've already examined these as they relate to OCD and anxiety; they can apply to depression too. You might experience our old friends **Catastrophising** or **Jumping To Conclusions**. So you might say, 'Oh, I can't be bothered going to the pool today; it's absolutely pointless as I won't enjoy it at all.' If that's what you think, you are unlikely to attempt to go swimming at all.

A better way of examining such a statement is to subject it to questioning:

1. Is it **100 per cent true** there is no point going to the swimming pool whatsoever?

   No, as I haven't even done it yet so I don't know what the outcome will be.

2. Is it **helpful** to think about it this way?

   No, because it's stopping me doing things.

If you answer 'no' to either of these questions, that opens up the possibility of looking at the situation another way. Perhaps you can say to yourself, 'OK, I have some bad days but friends tell me I'm making progress. So maybe a little swimming every week won't hurt.'

Again, we can use the '**One Hand**' and the '**Other Hand**' ways of interpreting. You can choose to go with your first explanation – but you can also choose to see it a different way too; a way that might be a truer representation of the reality of the situation. You can ask yourself:

> **Is this 100 per cent accurate?**
>
> **Is this a helpful way to think?**
>
> **Are there any thinking problems in my thoughts?**
>
> **Is there another way I can see this situation (on the other hand ...)?**

Remember, you don't have to make the new way of thinking about it sound perfect, because life is not perfect and often things can be difficult. You can reflect this in your new way of thinking; for example:

I know I am feeling low and it is really hard work getting to the pool, but there is a chance I will enjoy it even a little which is probably worth the huge effort to go!

DEPRESSION: SUMMARY

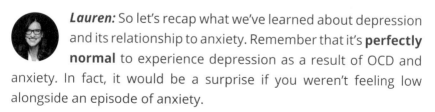 *Lauren:* So let's recap what we've learned about depression and its relationship to anxiety. Remember that it's **perfectly normal** to experience depression as a result of OCD and anxiety. In fact, it would be a surprise if you weren't feeling low alongside an episode of anxiety.

Depression has a number of symptoms, and while we may all experience some of these symptoms from time to time, if you have had low mood consistently for the past two weeks, and at least five of the other symptoms we discussed, then you are probably depressed.

Would you benefit from anti-depression medication? A lot of medication used to treat anxiety by medical specialists is also prescribed for depression, and it might be useful to speak with a medical specialist to consider this option. This could provide the boost you need as the sufferer of depression and anxiety; the step that allows you to start getting better.

However, medication isn't wholly necessary to make a recovery from depression. A good course of evidence-based treatment, to treat the anxiety problem and depression, can also help alleviate depression. Sleep can be a major factor and a regular sleep pattern can really help, as can regular exercise, doing some activities you previously enjoyed, doing an activity that can bring a small sense of achievement and healthy eating. Avoid comfort foods, and substitute foods high in fat, sugar and salt with more healthy options.

Finding the motivation to begin regular exercise when you're depressed can be hard at first, but if you build it up from short periods (five to ten minutes is fine) you will notice a significant improvement in your mood.

If you are struggling with motivation as a result of depression, please try a **'Behaviour Booster'**. Look at the swimming pool example we've shown you, and see where you can make that little bit of extra effort. The rewards might only seem minimal at first, but as time goes on this will change and you will feel some enjoyment in doing this again.

You can also choose how to interpret related depression by using the 'Two Hands Theory' we have described elsewhere in the PTT approach. You can look at the explanations you give yourself for what happens in life and see how they fit with reality. You might find that the explanation you've been offering yourself doesn't quite fit, and other reasons may have more positive outcomes. These don't have to be perfect – nothing in life is – but if you give yourself permission to take a positive step, you will find it has beneficial results.

ADAM'S CONCLUSION: DEPRESSION

 Adam: I developed depression because of the anxiety and OCD I was suffering from, particularly during my acute stages of anxiety-based mental illness during adulthood. For me, it was a very scary situation because I'd experienced nothing like it before. It is like living underneath a permanent cloud; nothing matters, you have no appetite for life and your motivation is gone. I dreaded going to bed because I couldn't sleep at night, and would feel terrible the following day. Unsurprisingly, I began to feel anxious and panicky about the thought of having prolonged depression and never being able to get rid of it. The vicious cycle began to turn and the more I felt anxious, the worse the depression seemed to get.

I would 'scan' myself every morning to see how I was, and if I was feeling lousy I'd spend the day asking myself 'Why do I feel this way?' 'How can I fight it off?' Now I see I was doing the things which, instead of removing the depression, actually made it stronger. What I should have been doing – and what I eventually learned – was to simply accept and embrace all the bad feelings and down days. Instead of scanning myself and having these internal fights, I just accepted that I was feeling bad. I understood that my state of mind WOULD change, and by fighting it I was achieving nothing. Even when I couldn't sleep I just accepted I was tired, and tried to get on with the day. By accepting and embracing it, I eventually took control of it.

The other thing about co-morbid depression is that it will fade once you start accepting and embracing your OCD and anxiety. As you follow the PTT approach within this book, you will start to see and feel the benefits, and this will produce more positive thoughts which in turn will lessen the depression. The golden rule is: don't fight. Have the courage to accept your state of mind and embrace it by allowing in all the fears, anxieties and 'down' moments, just as you would when you allow all the good moments, nice thoughts and uplifting sensations to be accepted into your mind.

For more on depression and other mental health issues, please visit The Shaw Mind Foundation at www.shawmindfoundation.org.

PANIC ATTACKS

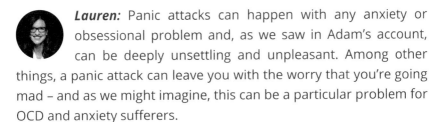 *Lauren:* Panic attacks can happen with any anxiety or obsessional problem and, as we saw in Adam's account, can be deeply unsettling and unpleasant. Among other things, a panic attack can leave you with the worry that you're going mad – and as we might imagine, this can be a particular problem for OCD and anxiety sufferers.

> What is a panic attack? Clinically it is described as **'an abrupt surge of intense fear or intense discomfort that reaches a peak within minutes.'** During that time, **four** (or more) of the following symptoms can occur:[22]
>
> • palpitations
> • sweating
> • trembling and shaking
> • shortness of breath
> • feelings of choking
> • chest pain
> • nausea or abdominal distress
> • dizziness
> • numbness
> • fear of losing control or going crazy
> • fear of dying.

All in all, a pretty unpleasant list, and anyone who has experienced a panic attack will know just how fear-inducing and debilitating they are. They can be expected or unexpected, they can occur during the day or at night and they can easily turn into a vicious cycle similar to the ones we've discussed elsewhere in this book.

22 American Psychiatric Association. (2013). *Diagnostic and Statistical Manual of Mental Disorders* (5th ed.). Washington, DC: American Psychiatric Association.

Below is a cognitive model of panic attacks, which we have reproduced with the permission of the author, Professor David Clark.[23]

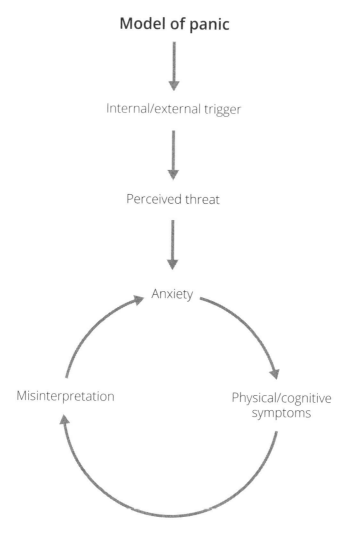

Figure 22: *Cognitive model of panic.*

As we can see, the attack is started by an internal or external trigger. You might feel a physical sensation – a tingling in your hands, your heart rate increasing, a feeling of shakiness – and because you've had those physiological reactions your **interpretation of events** is that it is in some way **catastrophic**. This is related to the symptoms you're

23 Clark, D. M. (1986). A cognitive approach to panic. *Behaviour Research and Therapy*, 24(4), 461–70.

experiencing, so it might be that you think you're having a heart attack, that you will lose control of your bladder and bowels, that you will faint or choke, or that you will go mad. These interpretations (or misinterpretations) then make you anxious, which in turn increases the physiological symptom severity and thus completes the vicious cycle and continues to make the anxiety and physical symptoms much worse.[24]

However, what is happening in your body is completely normal. Increased heart rate, shortness of breath, feeling hot and sweaty, blurry vision, sensations of choking and tingling feelings etc. are all signs that your body is going into primitive 'fight, flight or freeze' mode in response to a perceived threat. The irony is that the perceived threat is actually coming from you, because your body is in 'fight, flight or freeze' threat mode!

Of course, it's easy to say that such symptoms are completely normal. It doesn't feel that way at all when you're experiencing them, which is why people go to great lengths to avoid situations which might bring on a panic attack. Sufferers commonly carry around items which they hope will help in the event of an attack: paper bags, bottles of water, Valium, rescue remedies and other medication. This, of course, reinforces the belief that something dangerous is going on and, in a similar vein, sufferers may also avoid drinking fluids or going too far from a toilet, in case they lose control of their bodily functions.

You might remember how I treated Adam for panic attacks – after explaining the theory as I have done here, I then asked him to try his best to bring one on. At first he found this thought to be a fearful one, but try as he might he wasn't able to induce a panic attack at that very moment. So in effect, I was asking him to **embrace** the idea of a panic attack by going straight to the worry and proactively asking it to do its worst. Instead of avoiding the situation we do the opposite and **pull the trigger on the fear**. Obviously, I will only ask the sufferer to do this once they've understood thinking problems and the vicious

24   Clark, D. M., (1989) Anxiety states: Panic and generalized anxiety. In Hawton, Keith (Ed); Salkovskis, Paul M. (Ed); Kirk, Joan (Ed); Clark, David M. (Ed), (1989). *Cognitive Behaviour Therapy for Psychiatric Problems: A Practical Guide. Oxford Medical Publications* (pp. 52–96). New York, NY, US: Oxford University Press.

cycle of panic attacks, and how to accept their OCD and anxiety. If you've understood and absorbed that, you're in a good position to try an **embrace** technique for panic attacks.

Challenging and changing the interpretation of the physiological symptoms is an effective way of helping to deal with panic attacks. Let's look at a typical belief that, as a result of a panic attack, you will go mad:

> **Q: How many times have you had a panic attack in the past year?**
>
> A: Approximately ten times per month.
>
> **Q: So that's approximately 120 panic attacks this year?**
>
> A: Yes, that's right.
>
> **Q: Have you gone mad?**
>
> A: No.
>
> **Q: Have you been sectioned or committed to a psychiatric hospital?**
>
> A: No.
>
> **Q: Has life gone back to normal following the attack?**
>
> A: Yes.
>
> **Q: How many people do you know have gone mad through panic attacks?**
>
> A: None.

So based on this evidence, the truth is that it is very unlikely that you will go mad as a result of a panic attack. In addition, if you haven't gone mad but you've had over 120 panic attacks, it is probably unlikely that it will happen the next time.

We can also subject this to the **'One Hand/Other Hand'** test, in that:

On the 'One Hand' I feel I will pass out or have a heart attack …

On the 'Other Hand' my body is going through a natural 'fight, flight or freeze' process and while I find it very uncomfortable, it is in fact a normal experience and not dangerous, and will pass soon

Evidence for this position being true: my heart rate is going so fast it must be unnatural and therefore a sign I am having a heart attack.

Evidence for this position being true:
- I have had over 120 panic attacks over the past six months and I've never had a heart attack.
- In addition, panic attacks are an anxiety response, anxiety is a normal human experience that everyone goes through in life, and not everyone who experiences anxiety then has a heart attack (in fact, panic attacks are not known as a trigger for heart attacks!)

> Based on the evidence, panic attacks are short episodes of intense anxiety. Although unpleasant and annoying, panic attacks are not dangerous.

Table 19: Example of using on the One Hand and on the Other Hand method to challenge panic attacks.

You can also see the problematic thinking patterns that we discussed earlier at play here. The person suffering from panic attacks **catastrophises** their symptoms and makes it a 'worst case' scenario. But, as we know, problematic thinking patterns contribute to the cycle of anxiety and prevent us from embracing and challenging the situations in which we feel anxious.

When I was a student I once spent a whole night working on an assignment that had to be handed in the following day. I barely slept and drank a lot of coffee. The following morning I had a panic attack on the way in to the university. But I didn't see this as a threat that I was going mad or having a heart attack. My interpretation was that I'd been up all night working, fuelled by coffee and that my body was reacting in a normal way. The sensations weren't pleasant but they soon passed and I was able to carry on as normal. My interpretation was not catastrophic and my experience had been unpleasant yet normal and would pass. This allowed me to step aside from the vicious cycle of panic.

There are some more common catastrophic interpretations that people have during panic attacks. These include going mad, having a heart attack, fainting or passing out, losing control of body functions, choking and suffocating. This list is not exhaustive, and there are numerous other catastrophic interpretations that people may have, so just because your main fear is not mentioned here, that does not mean it is not a panic attack! You can challenge your catastrophic interpretation in the same way, whatever your feared outcome is.

Changing the interpretation is vital. It allows you to accept and embrace the panic attack, and let the feelings be without avoiding the triggers that bring them on. Indeed, those triggers should be actively sought out so that you're carrying out exposure experiments, just as we've shown you with OCD and anxiety. Until you actively embrace them, you will not get on top of panic attacks and they will continue to be fearful and dangerous for as long as you let them.

Just like the OCD and other anxiety problems, our behaviour also has a role to play so also needs to be challenged. Remember in the OCD section how Adam had a number of behaviours that he used to keep himself 'safe', but that in fact reinforced the OCD. As we mentioned above, the same thing happens during panic attacks – people use a number of behaviours designed to protect themselves from the feared consequence. As with OCD, avoidance is a big part of these behaviours. For example, someone who worries they might go mad from a panic attack will go to extreme lengths to avoid feeling anxious, including avoiding watching scary movies, avoiding going anywhere new or busy, ensuring they always have someone with them when they leave the house and carrying anti-anxiety tablets with them at all times, 'just in case'. However, now we know that panic attacks are a normal but unpleasant human experience, these behaviours are unnecessary and preventing the person from finding out that in fact they won't go mad if they have a panic attack. These behaviours are also a burden and will reduce the quality of life of the person suffering from panic attacks. Avoidance and 'safe' behaviours can take many forms and are anything that a person believes 'prevents' them or 'protects' them from having a panic attack.

In order to identify the things you are avoiding and the 'safe' behaviours you have put in place, ask yourself:

What are the things I have stopped doing in case I have a panic attack?

E.g., using trains and buses, watching scary movies, going for my morning jog, drinking water before a meeting etc.

What places have I stopped visiting in case I have a panic attack?

E.g., any place that I think might be busy, any place in which I have to queue, any place that I can't 'escape' quickly, any place that I don't know where the toilets are.

What things have I started doing to make sure I don't have a panic attack?

E.g., carrying water and a paper bag with me everywhere I go, ensuring that I always have someone with me when I leave the house, taking taxis rather than public transport, making sure I know where the bathrooms are whenever I go anywhere, making sure I have my phone and emergency numbers programmed in my mobile phone.

After you have changed the interpretation and identified the things you are avoiding and your 'safe' behaviours, we have to do what we did previously with the OCD and anxiety where we **embraced** the situation. So you might now understand rationally that panic attacks are unpleasant, distressing but ultimately harmless events. However, you now need to embrace the situation in which they occur, whether it be a stand-alone event or as part of another problem. Using the same structure we used earlier in embracing the OCD, you need to embrace the panic attacks and set yourself some experiments to test out whether the catastrophic interpretation is true or your new revised interpretations.

My catastrophic interpretation is ...
that if I have a panic attack, I will go mad.

What does the evidence say?
- Panic attacks are extreme episodes of anxiety but are not dangerous and will not make me go mad.

My experiment is:
- Allow myself to have a panic attack if it happens and not use any of my safety behaviours. I will go to somewhere I have avoided out of worry that I might have a panic attack. Therefore, I will go to the park on my own for twenty minutes without carrying my phone.

Outcome of my experiment:
- I felt very anxious and felt a panic attack coming on when I was at the park, but I stayed in the park and eventually it passed. It was very unpleasant and scary, but I am in one piece and I didn't go mad.

What can I do to build on this experiment?
- I can go to the park for longer next time. I could also take a bus for one or two stops as I have been avoiding taking the bus.

Table 20: *Example experiment sheet for embracing panic attacks.*

Now fill in the box below ...

My catastrophic interpretation is ...

_____

What does the evidence say?

_____

_____

My experiment is to ...

_____

_____

_____

_____

Outcome of my experiment:

_____

_____

What can I do to build on this experiment?

_____

_____

_____

Table 21: *Setting an experiment to embrace my panic attacks.*

It is important to remember that the goal is *not to not have a panic attack*. In embracing your panic attacks, you may experience one or even a few panic attacks. The goal is to challenge your catastrophic interpretation of what *might* happen should you either have a panic attack or be in the situation where you think you might have one.

When you start embracing the panic attacks, it might be easier to do it in gradual stages. For example, if you have been avoiding the bus or taking the train, you may want to start with taking the bus for two or three stops. Whether or not you have a panic attack, the next time do it three or four stops, and so on. If you have spent twenty minutes in a place that is very uncomfortable, the next time spend thirty minutes, the time after that forty-five minutes, and so on. It is important to continue to build on your progress too. You successfully took the bus two or three stops, so you need to push yourself each day and take the bus daily and for longer each time. If you do one experiment and think, 'Oh phew, I've done it now and nothing bad has happened, I'd better not push it', this is another way of avoiding and may even reinforce the panic attacks because you are still worried that the feared outcome might be true.

In embracing panic attacks, you will eventually find that you gain more control over your life, rather than your life being controlled by panic attacks and the avoidance and restrictions that come with them.

PANIC ATTACKS: SUMMARY

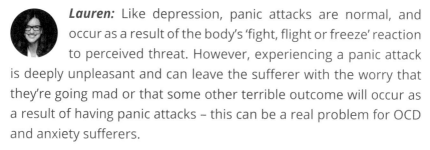

Lauren: Like depression, panic attacks are normal, and occur as a result of the body's 'fight, flight or freeze' reaction to perceived threat. However, experiencing a panic attack is deeply unpleasant and can leave the sufferer with the worry that they're going mad or that some other terrible outcome will occur as a result of having panic attacks – this can be a real problem for OCD and anxiety sufferers.

Panic attacks produce physical sensations – sweating, shaking, palpitations – which can make you think you're experiencing the symptoms of a serious illness or some other catastrophic outcome, such as a heart attack, losing control of your bladder, or fainting or losing control of yourself in other ways. These interpretations (or misinterpretations) then make you anxious, which in turn increases the physiological symptom severity and thus completes the vicious cycle, which continues to make the anxiety and physical symptoms much worse.

Challenging and changing the interpretation of the physiological symptoms is an effective first step in dealing with panic attacks. You can do this by employing the **Two Hands Theory**. For example, if you believe you might go mad, you can tell yourself either:

a) On the One Hand, I feel I will pass out, have a heart attack or go crazy,

or

b) On the Other Hand, my body is going through a natural 'fight, flight or freeze' process, and while I find it very uncomfortable, it is in fact a normal experience, not dangerous and will pass soon.

Changing the interpretation is vital. It allows you to accept and embrace the panic attack, and let the feelings be without avoiding the triggers that bring them on. Indeed, those triggers should be actively sought out so that you're carrying out exposure experiments, just as we've shown you with OCD and anxiety. When you've accepted this explanation, you can then go on to challenge and embrace panic attacks by attempting to bring one on, just like I did with Adam. Until you actively embrace them, you will not get on top of panic attacks, and they will continue to be fearful and dangerous for as long as you let them.

ADAM'S CONCLUSION: PANIC ATTACKS

 Adam: Panic attacks feel terrifying, to the point where you think you're going mad, like I did. The very thought of having one made me incredibly anxious, but what I didn't know at the time of my suffering was that they thrive on fear. When you're anticipating all the thoughts and sensations crowding in and attacking your mind and body, it's no wonder you're scared. Of course, the vicious cycle begins to spin and the situation becomes worse as you desperately try to fight off the panic attack. So how do you deal with a panic attack when you're in the thick of it? If you've been following the PTT approach, you can probably guess what I'm going to say next ... The simple way, and indeed the only way in my view, to deal with panic attacks is not to fight them but say yes, to accept and embrace what's going on.

Sounds easier said than done? Well, yes, to a certain extent. You need to find courage to allow a panic attack to happen, and even more courage to tell it to do its absolute worst. But if you do, you will see just how the fear will shrink as quickly as it arrived. Say to yourself, 'OK, I'm having a panic attack. There's no point fighting it, so I might as well let it come on and ask it to do its worst.' Now you've found the courage to face the attack, and by doing so you are embracing the whole experience, and lessening it each time you face it. You will still feel uncomfortable when a panic attack arrives, but the more you invite it in, the more you will reduce its power.

Instead of fearing it, call its bluff and tell it you are going to enjoy every moment and you want it to do its very worst; beg it to give you the worst panic attack that it has ever given you. As Lauren mentioned, eventually she asked me to try my very best to bring on a panic attack while we were parked up in the car, because I had a fear of having one while driving the kids somewhere. By this stage I'd accepted that I had panic attacks, but when I tried to bring one on, try as I might I simply couldn't do it at that particular moment. By accepting, I'd removed the fuel that powered the attack. Try it for yourself, and see what happens. You'll be surprised at how powerful you feel and how lacking in substance the panic attack actually is. I have never had a panic attack since.

Panic attacks may initially seem like a complex problem to us sufferers, but in my view – and once you take the step to face them head on – you will see that they are anything but complex.

In reality, panic attacks have no backbone, hold no special powers over us and are simply fuelled and supported by our own internal fear. We are the creator of our panic attacks and we are the source of all its fuel. That may be hard to believe at this stage, particularly if you are a sufferer currently going through the really unpleasant internal turmoil of suffering from panic and panic attacks, but it's 100 per cent accurate. The one and only thing a panic attack uses as its fuel is our own fear, which we give in abundance leading up to and during a panic attack. Cut off the fuel supply, and watch the intensity of the panic and panic attacks decrease!

So allowing ourselves to view panic and panic attacks as complex problems ensures we play further into the hands of our panic. It adds additional worry and fear which fuels and increases the perceived significance and importance of panic in our lives.

How do we break the cycle of panic attacks?

The answer is that we do this by simply taking a link out of the panic cycle chain. This link is fear. Again, this sounds easier said than done, right? Well, to some extent this is true, because taking fear out of the equation is achieved by facing our fears head-on and as we know, challenging our fears is initially very hard to do. It takes courage; the same amount of courage that is needed to take your life back from the other mental health issues such as OCD and anxiety which we have discussed in this book. Our recovery approach technique – **Accept, Embrace and Control** – is a really effective way of dealing with our panic and panic attacks. We don't fight the panic attack, we accept it and we have the courage to face it head-on by embracing the panic attack in all its glory. In doing so we take control, and panic no longer dictates to us how we live our lives. Show the panic that you are willing to accept and embrace it – anytime, anywhere – and in doing so, you will cut off its fuel supply which it so desperately needs and relies on.

However, you need to remember not to fall into the trap of just telling yourself to accept and embrace by simply saying those words. Instead, allow yourself to go through the process of really feeling all the emotions and sensations that come with letting in all the panic and panic attacks, and do it without compromise, allowing them to be there for as long as they want to.

In short, open the door and go straight to the source. It is very frightening at first and it feels really uncomfortable. It will also feel counter-productive to you at first as your instinct will immediately be to fight, run away or do anything to stop or ease the panic. But remember that running away or fighting has the opposite effect in trying to eliminate your panic attacks because such reactions just reinforce the sensation that there is something to be afraid of, and therefore we unwittingly provide the panic with the fuel it needs to thrive, through the fear we give it. Instead, **accept** and **embrace**; doing this will allow you to be in **control** of your mental health, including panic attacks.

SECTION 5

FITNESS AND DIET

Adam: We have never wanted this book and PTT approach to be one of prescription. We try hard not to say 'You must do this' or 'You have to do that'. Our survival and recovery approach is definitive, but we can only ever advise – we can't compel you as the sufferer to do anything. This section about fitness and diet is based on my own personal experience, and it may be that presently you don't feel well enough to take up the advice offered in this section. That's completely understandable, but I would ask you not to completely dismiss it. At first I was extremely sceptical of the benefits that exercise and a change in diet might give me, but after making such changes I had to rethink my attitude. So please read on, with an open mind!

As you might remember from my personal story in Part I, I was a very sporty boy, and that continued as I became a teenager and beyond. I loved sport and still do; the problem was that as anxiety took hold I stopped focusing on my body and instead concentrated on the workings of my mind – which of course did me no good at all. I went from being tall and skinny to being tall and overweight. In the period leading up to my most acute episode of OCD I was 18 stones (250 lbs) and getting bigger. In short, I'd just stopped looking after myself properly and could barely be bothered to get out of bed. I was tired and severely drained mentally, which seemed to have zapped all my physical energy away.

I see now that this was the related depression which almost invariably comes with an anxiety problem such as OCD. These days, when we're all so busy and very time-poor, cramming in an hour to concentrate on exercise is hard enough, but when you're depressed as well, it seems even more of a huge mountain to climb. So you just turn away from it and head for the sofa, the takeaway and the cans of sugary soda; nice, comforting things that will temporarily take away or at the very least ease your pain and misery.

It's a classic image – the overweight, depressed person lying on the sofa or in bed, too down and demotivated to move any further than the fridge. But that was the person I was becoming and after I had my third and worst crash, and subsequently met Lauren, I resolved to do something about it.

After a couple of sessions with Lauren I started to look more closely at OCD, anxiety and related depression, and on forum after forum on the internet, I noticed how people talked about exercise as a way of keeping it at bay – the depression part, at least. I was sceptical. The first doctor I saw about my problems all those years ago told me to 'go and have a nice walk in the park', as though that would magically cure the severe anxiety I was experiencing. It's all very well for doctors and fitness experts telling those with mental health issues to go out and exercise – if they could walk a day in our shoes, with all our anguish and suffering, they'd soon understand how challenging even a simple activity can be.

There was another problem too. I realised that taking exercise, particularly of the cardio-vascular kind, would increase my adrenalin levels and possibly keep my anxiety spinning. I was terrified of doing anything that would bring on yet another panic attack. So I was both demotivated and fearful, and yet I realised I had to do something to stop myself becoming even more sluggish and out of shape. Now I know that exercise was actually the perfect way to **embrace** the anxiety and panic (as in, bring it on as an experiment), as well as having its own natural benefits.

What I needed was a touch of courage, the same courage I had to locate in order to accept and embrace my anxiety. I had to dig deep and find the last remains of energy and strength I had to motivate myself to do something. I was so poorly at that stage that when we tried to take the kids to a theme park, we had to come straight home because I couldn't find the energy or the courage to even get out of the car.

The feeling I had though after meeting Lauren was one of hope. Only a little bit, but that was enough. No matter how bad or poorly we feel, we all have it within ourselves to find that little bit of hope and therefore motivation. So I began an exercise 'programme', which was barely worthy of the name as it consisted of two twenty-minute walks, up the road and back, every day. It sounds easy but believe me, it was one of the toughest things I ever had to do. The morning walk was the worst because my anxiety and depression were at their height then and just the thought of getting out of bed seemed an impossible task. Still, I pushed on, hoping with my little bit of hope and my newfound approach of facing the fear that I would feel marginally better.

And, after five days doing this, I did notice a change. It was a small one, admittedly, and it came in the form of almost looking forward to the walks, even the morning one. The sense of dread I felt had started to dissipate and there was just a hint of motivation in my first steps out of the door. Something was telling me to stay on track, even though I was still very poorly. The sensation was similar to the one you feel when you're on a diet. The first few days are really tough as your mind tells you to give up and go back to the comforting junk food you've been shovelling down. If you get through this bit, those thoughts lessen and begin to be replaced by more positive ones, especially when you start to notice the physical changes.

At the time I really should've given myself a pat on the back for having the motivation to stick at it for a week. As small as the progress is, it is really important to recognise and positively reinforce any minor improvements you see in yourself during a recovery. However, the nature of my illness meant that I was shut off from positive thoughts; to find and give myself encouragement felt pointless. I shuffled up and down that road like a zombie, hardly daring to believe that it might be helping in some way.

Moving into my second week of exercise, I summoned the courage and strength to include a short jogging session into one of the daily walks. Although this was hard, I had to remind myself that the previous week I'd been almost suicidal as I left the house and couldn't fathom surviving the next minute, let alone the next day or a week.

Now I was in my second week of exercise, which included a short jog. The next couple of weeks saw me replace my walking routine entirely with moderate jogging.

This was very tough. The additional adrenalin pumping through my body raised my anxiety levels even further. I had very little energy, and there were days when I cried because the energy to jog just didn't seem to be there and my anxiety was soaring. I'd come back home and feel weak, then I'd cry even more because I felt even worse than I did before I set off; it just felt like I was going backwards in terms of recovery and I found it really upsetting. Even so, the hope still burned in me and three weeks into my exercise plan I had a routine. This was now beginning to look like progress, because previously I'd had no routine other than lying in bed. My mental health wasn't much better – I was still suffering with strong OCD urges, anxiety and depression – but my attitude had begun to turn into one that said, 'I am now on a positive track, and I will and I am going to get my life back.'

Furthermore, I was beginning to develop pleasure from getting fit and doing moderate exercise. I noticed that rather than feeling worse after getting back from my run, I had a new sense of relaxation and calm. This gave me further hope and helped me maintain my exercise routine. Whenever I had a day where I wanted to skip my exercise, I would simply remind myself that I would feel much better with the uplifting sensation that came from the exercise after the run.

A month into my exercise plan, I now understood why all the specialists within the mental health industry promote a healthy and active lifestyle. It is certainly not a miracle cure or a key to everlasting positive mental health, but regular exercise gives you the tools and armour you need to deal with mental health issues, even those of a severe nature. It provides you with energy, focus, patience and, more importantly, motivation to challenge your demons.

A parallel issue to the one of exercise was my eating habits. As I said, I ballooned in weight, caused by a diet of junk food and sugary drinks. I simply couldn't be bothered to eat properly and had gone into the classic depressive's 'pick-me-up' remedy, eating comfort foods high in fat, sugar and starch. Comfort eating provides a relatively short-term fix and works on the same principle as entering the vicious cycle of anxiety in that the more you do to distract yourself, the faster the cycle turns. So something had to change.

Luckily, 'cutting down' doesn't mean 'cutting out'. These foods were a pleasure in my life, and to take them away entirely would have made me even more depressed because it was the only minor pleasure I was experiencing in my life at the time. So I decided on a common-sense approach, in that I would balance my diet with more vegetables, fish, pulses, fruit smoothies, salad and rice, and have a bit of what I really enjoyed a couple of times a week. It was important to have something to look forward to in the week, and actually it became a motivating factor for me to keep going with the exercise routine. I swapped soda and beer for water, and at the weekends or on occasions allowed myself to let my hair down a little and have a sugary drink, or a glass or two of wine and some tasty, hearty comfort food.

The weekends became my reward, and my goal to work towards, and each weekend I wanted to see an improvement in myself from the previous weekend. My fitness and diet had changed dramatically over the last six weeks and I'd lost around one and a half stone (21 lbs) in weight. Some of this, I admit, was down to a loss of appetite due to depression but hope was now growing – if I could achieve all this in six weeks, when I was so close to suicide, then what could I achieve in the next six weeks and beyond? 'Is it possible I could get some form of life back?' I asked myself. 'Is it possible I could even fully recover?' I was by no means cured of my illness, but had indeed found myself in a place where, for the very first time in my life, I felt I had the motivation and increased hope that maybe I might have the strength to tackle my OCD, anxiety and depression. Every cloud has a silver lining and mental illness actually gave me my motivation back through achieving fitness.

You can recover from an anxiety-based mental illness like OCD without taking up exercise, but I can say that exercising gave me a platform to deal with the issues I was having. As Lauren might put it, those twenty-minute walks which turned into jogs were a 'helpful distraction' that enabled me to motivate myself towards accepting, embracing and eventually controlling my OCD and anxiety. And yes, you can ALWAYS find time to exercise, even if you're the busiest person on the planet. A twenty-minute walk costs nothing, and it's never, ever a waste of time.

In conclusion, if any of the above has struck a chord with you and you feel that exercise might bring some benefit into your life, then please find that little bit of hope within you to get up, get out and take a breath of a fresh air. You don't have to approach it like you're training for a marathon. Start slowly and simply, and build up gradually. I promise that you will be amazed by what you can achieve. And don't be too hard on yourself – remember how Lauren asks us to treat ourselves with compassion – but as far as you can, stick with it. Looking after yourself physically is a kind and compassionate thing to do for yourself. In the long term it will bring so many rewards and benefits. To conclude, *I firmly believe that there isn't a challenge that exists that can rival the strength of the determined human spirit. I believe this because I am also proof of it.*

SECTION 6

FAMILY AND FRIENDS

When They Should Help the OCD and Anxiety Sufferer – And When They Really Shouldn't ...

Adam: In this book and the PTT approach, we've touched several times on the subject of friends and family in relation to the OCD and anxiety sufferer. My family were supportive of me, but, like most families, didn't really understand OCD and anxiety and what underpins it. I don't blame them for this in any way – anxiety-related disorders are very slippery indeed and it's difficult enough for the sufferer to get a handle on them, never mind their nearest and dearest. Professional understanding and help is needed, which is why we decided to write this book and invest in the resources to make this approach readily available on a global scale.

As we've said, friends and relatives can be supportive and understanding of our situation and in many ways they can help practically as we're following the PTT approach. What they CAN'T do is reassure the sufferer in a way that keeps the anxiety going. This is a really hard thing because reassurance is what parents, partners and friends tend to do when you're in trouble – 'Don't worry, it'll all work out fine, you'll see' etc. That's fine for many things in life, but for anxiety it works the opposite way, in that it just helps to keep it going.

Perhaps the best perspective of the relationship between an anxiety sufferer and their loved ones should come from someone close to the sufferer, and so I'm very pleased that Alissa, my wife, has agreed to provide an account of my problems with OCD and anxiety from her perspective. Alissa will give families and sufferers an insight into the difficulties faced by loved ones, as well as sound advice about learning to manage such difficulties in a domestic setting without reassuring and helping to continue the problem ...

Alissa Shaw: Adam and I first met when I was just born and he was a five-year-old boy. I couldn't yet hold my own head up, and he was already beginning his journey through a life with OCD. Our parents are close friends, so we spent a bit of time together growing up, although the age and gender difference kept us at a distance until I reached 17, when we both realised our feelings had changed and grown.

As I grew closer to Adam I never saw anything unusual in his behaviour. He was actually the most relaxed, easy-going, happy person I'd ever come to know. I'd no idea what was happening underneath that. He clearly liked to focus and work hard, but he certainly didn't appear stressed or worried much of the time and he was fun to be around.

Soon into our relationship, our first daughter was born. It was a difficult time for us, as she was born with a condition called talipes, known as 'clubbed foot'. It meant many regular hospital visits and surgery so it was a distressing thing for us to deal with. However, Adam never seemed phased by any of this and coped very well throughout. It brought us closer together and we came through it as a team.

I had absolutely no idea that Adam had difficulties around his thoughts. He showed no signs and had no obvious habits. He didn't say a single word to me until we were in Lanzarote on our first vacation together as a family, when the first episode occurred. I remember him being in our room extremely upset. I went in to see him and he was just repeating, 'I'm not well, I'm not well.' I was totally bewildered and equally terrified. My initial thoughts were, 'He's seeing someone else or he's seriously ill.' I didn't know what to think, but as he explained as best he could, I tried to understand it. He didn't have a clue himself about what was happening to him. I didn't have a clue about OCD or anxiety.

There seemed to be no triggering factor for Adam. He was in a salaried job and was doing fine, and we were happy together. It just seemed to come from nowhere. Adam isn't the type to cry easily, so I just reassured him, trying to make him feel better. I wanted to comfort him, which is human nature. I admit it worried me, in that I thought, 'Is this just how it will be from now on?' Of course I love Adam deeply so this was something we were going to get through together.

On our wedding day a couple of years later, I felt proud of how far we'd come, and 'for better or worse' couldn't have felt more true … I had no idea how much more was to come …

When he started to build the business it became more serious. Adam rapidly changed and deteriorated. That's when I thought, 'This is actually very bad.' He couldn't get out of bed. It was a dreadful time. I thought he may never get out of bed again and this was how our lives would be.

Day-to-day life was hard, both in a practical sense and emotionally, on all of us. During this time I had to work half-days as I couldn't leave Adam alone for any longer than this. He would spend the entire day in his room unable to face anything or anyone.

There were occasions which were especially difficult. Our daughter's birthday was particularly sad for us, as Adam spent the day at his parents' house and couldn't make the party. Situations like that can make it all even harder to understand and be understanding.

I believe that in order for us, as relatives or friends of someone with anxiety, to remain supportive and always caring and understanding towards that loved one, we have to understand as much as we can about the illness and how it is affecting them. So read and understand but also communicate and discuss as much as you can together. This can be very helpful to those concerned. Once when I was having a particularly bad day, Adam said to me:

'You can still talk to me you know. Yes, I'm having a really bad time, but I still love and care about you just the same.'

And so I would communicate with him how I was feeling. That small element of normality helped me, but also helped Adam to regain some confidence in himself and his progress.

Of course, small steps were necessary in building this back up. We took small trips out on the days he felt capable, to a local shop or something simple.

Something to remember here is that one trip out one day can be quite a success but the next can be not so good at all. I found that a little disheartening at times, but I realised that this is perfectly OK and I learnt to accept the 'up and down' nature of Adam's recovery.

When Adam started seeing his first therapist, Michael, it was like we had been thrown a lifeline. He started to have a little more positivity again, which helped me to feel more positive too. It gave me a huge amount of hope. Even so, he was still very unwell and it was very frustrating when I just needed a day of 'normal'. I was trying to deal with everything and it was a constant strain; you can't think about anything else because it's there all of the time. You can sometimes feel as though there's no escape from this new way of life that has been thrown upon you.

In his first therapy sessions, Adam started to get his personality back. I saw there was hope, and at the end of the time that he had with his first therapist we really thought, 'We've nailed this. It's done. Never again.' I presumed that because we had the diagnosis of OCD and because of the therapy Adam went through, I could put this part of our lives safely to the back of my mind.

He went back to work and felt more positive, and I supported him when he wanted to put everything into his new business.

The impact of heavy work can be hard on a partner and it was often lonely when Adam was working long hours and I only had the kiddies for company, but Adam was happy working hard. It's just in his make-up and as the rewards came, these things made it worthwhile.

As he's described, Adam's OCD came back when the 'just fear' mantra he developed from his first therapist didn't seem to work for him any more. He was quite good at keeping the signs from me; he didn't want to drop that on me again. I really didn't see it coming.

Now though, I would most likely see the signs. You learn to spot the little details, the routines developing. Over the years I've tried to recognise which things are 'normal' and the things which mean we need to have a 'chat'. Even today he still has some rare but very minor and funny little things, like how he washes and applies cream. Occasionally I will gently mix up his routines, to test his response. For example, after he's dried his hands with a tea towel he always likes to put it next to the sink, so I will say, 'You need to put that back properly because it won't dry.' If I sense any anxiety from him, which these days is now very rare, I know we may need a chat. If not, that's great.

It's the same with one of our daughters who is much like Adam in many ways. Her routines and rituals are more obvious, but they may not be to other people. I do similar things with her. She has a lot of little routines and rituals which really do trouble her so we have to keep on top of that. The latest thing was her checking her bed, under her duvet, mattress, pillows, under the towel, in the window for spiders. She's checking, checking, checking.

Sometimes she has a bit of a blinking or swallowing thing. Sometimes we just watch to see how she's swallowing her food. We have a 'worries list' for her and a chart, to help her through her anxieties. It can be very distressing to see anxiety in your child, and it can be emotionally draining at times.

A positive to come out of Adam's illness and his recovery is that we are acutely aware of the signs and are therefore able to give any of our children the very best support if we feel issues around their mental health well-being ever need addressing. We are very lucky in that sense, as there's nothing worse than seeing your child suffer, either physically or mentally, and be unable to help them. I know Adam is very thankful for this and says he would go through the whole process again just for the knowledge he has acquired, which has given us the ability to support our children's mental health well-being now and in the future if ever required. He remembers all too well the pain and suffering he went through as a child.

What continues to drive him forward now is the prevention of this happening to our own children, and children and adult sufferers around the world. I believe there's always a positive to come out of a negative, no matter how bad the negative.

It's hard for any parent or partner of a sufferer. You want to comfort that person but you can't. It's natural to reassure someone close to us who is anxious, but with OCD and anxiety you just can't do that. The main thing is to be aware. Watch for the signs. Be prepared to step in and ask if any behaviour worries you.

At this point I would also like to mention Adam's fears of hurting others mentioned throughout this book. Of course, if you previously have little knowledge about OCD this can be hard to hear at first, and you may have wondered what it means, as I did. But that never worried me, in a sense of, 'Oh no, what if he actually does something like that?' I knew him too well and I knew that that was OK for someone suffering with OCD and anxiety … we know that he was anxious because it's something he would never want to do.

The last severe OCD episode for Adam was the worst yet. We were living in Lanzarote and enjoying the lifestyle. Adam was working back in the UK for a few days and I called him to tell him that my lovely granddad had passed away. I was so upset I couldn't get any words out and Adam immediately panicked because he thought something had happened to the kids. At that point he just lost it. He couldn't cope with the worry of us being alone there, with him in the UK. I think the panic and anxiety built up and eventually he was at crisis point again. I remember him saying, 'I need to get an apartment, I need to stay at home and get better.' He soon reached a stage where he couldn't get out of bed again. All I could do was speak with him over the phone but he could barely reply.

He was a wreck. He would say things like, 'I can't think straight. I feel like I'm dying. I can't get these thoughts out of my mind. I will never get better this time.' That was all I could get out of him – the fear he wouldn't get better. It was OCD about OCD. It gets very complicated, especially trying to figure out the right responses and thinking before you speak. It can be like speaking a foreign language; you have to think before you know what to say, and it's like that when speaking to a loved one with OCD. As you've read, reassurance seeking can be tricky and persistent! So don't be caught out! I found the best way to respond was either with a little humour; for example, if Adam was asking 'What if I don't get better?' I would say, 'Adam, stop asking silly questions or I will get tough in a minute!!'

Or I would use a simple but kind response such as, 'Adam, we will get through this together and you're doing so well.' Sometimes diverting the conversation is another way of avoiding reassurance.

And so I had to pack up in Lanzarote and take the kids out of school. Adam's mum came over to help me bring them back to the UK. It was a horrible time and I just wanted to be back with Adam. It was the longest we had ever been apart and I missed him, but I knew I'd be going home to someone with a lot of problems.

Back home I explained to the kids that daddy was having bad headaches. It was complicated to explain and they were too young to understand. They weren't in school because they'd just about finished for summer and we were now living in the countryside. I had to be home with the kids every day and be around for Adam, making sure he ate and drank, and I didn't want him to be alone. It was tough on the kids; they missed having daddy to play with or chat to, and it was hard on Adam too, feeling he couldn't do these things.

For several weeks the kids 'lost' their daddy and I 'lost' my husband and best friend once again. I actually think that was the hardest thing of all. Adam is the person I would always turn to in difficulty and he was also the person I would chat with and have a laugh with. So for a while, life was a struggle.

I was also worried his business would fail. It was doing very well but he had to be there running it, and there were several points when I thought he would never get back to it. What would we do then? It bothered me, not in a way that we wouldn't have money any more, but more like, 'How the heck are we going to manage?' And I knew Adam wouldn't be happy going back to a salaried job as an employee. It was chaos: that's the best way to describe those few weeks.

That episode lasted several weeks, then he found Lauren. We were very fortunate to have the resources to pay for private help and in turn Adam was able to receive this help and support in the form of a very talented and supportive therapist. I remember her saying, 'Adam, we can have you better in a few weeks. We are going to approach this in a way that you've never tried before, and it will work.' The relief I felt at that moment was incredible. We put our faith in her totally and I knew she excelled in her field. I felt like I had someone on my side finally. Her coming into our lives, having her help, and knowing it was the right help this time, was just fantastic.

All I did at that first meeting was sit and listen to Adam and Lauren talk. She explained about the reassurance and not doing it and described in a simple way how OCD works so that I could understand it too. She was just lovely. We owe her so much because I simply do not know where we would be now without her.

After four weeks of therapy we took our first outing as a family. Adam really struggled but this was about him embracing his anxiety and he knew it was part of his recovery. He was fearful of other people and of breaking down in front of them. It was now about getting him slowly used to the outside world again.

Lauren was spot on about the recovery time. We were on a good path and this time it felt like we'd really got it. From there we could start to think about the future and we decided to have another child. It was a positive and a new chapter of our lives, and so we were expecting child number five! It was a sweet ending to a very difficult period.

Despite a lot of pain, Adam's OCD has played some part in his success. He says that himself and I agree. I remember Lauren saying that a lot of successful people have OCD. I think that's very interesting. I would never take that part of his personality away, despite the bad times it has caused. It's part of who he is and I too feel I've certainly grown in strength from the entire experience.

If you are a family member or friend reading this I would say, 'Remember to look after yourself through all of this.' That sounds obvious but it's easy to forget.

And it's OK to turn to other people for support, whether that be someone close to you or a new person. But I think in this situation it's a good idea to speak with your loved one before doing so. I know in my case Adam didn't want me to discuss what was happening with people close to us until he had it all figured out. He soon realised, however, that there was no reason to feel embarrassed or ashamed and that actually what he has been through, what we have been through together, shows real strength.

Throughout the recovery time I frequently wanted to ask Adam, 'How are you today? How are you feeling? Are you not so good today?' This is something I quickly learnt to avoid, as it then made Adam scan himself and do checks to see what answer to give me. So I found it helpful to make a list of appropriate comments to show Adam that I was thinking about him and caring, such as, 'I hope you slept OK last night' or 'I bet it was hard to jog out in the rain today; you did well!' If I was ever stuck with what to say, a simple gesture, such as a hug, always filled the space perfectly.

My final piece of advice is that all people who are close to your loved one, such as friends and family, need to be in on this too. They need to do the same as you, otherwise they could dole out reassurance and, without realising, undo your hard work. It's also good to encourage normality between these people and your loved one. They need to behave and converse as they always did, but it's important to have that chat about giving no reassurance so that you can all follow these rules together. Adam used to call his mum sometimes to get some level of reassurance from her, but after I explained this to her she quickly got the hang of it. Everybody was very supportive of this.

To all of you reading this book as friends and relatives going through this difficult time with the sufferer: although it may seem relentless, exhausting or overwhelming at times, and even if your life as it was is unrecognisable, remember that this won't last forever. Just as I'm writing this today, you will look back on this time with greater strength. I wish you the very best on your journey there. Recovery, even in the most severe cases, is achievable; Adam is a perfect example of this.

Pulling the Trigger, Juniors and Teenagers Edition, including guidance for parents, is also available. Please visit www.pulling-the-trigger.com

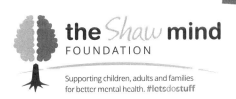

the *Shaw* mind
FOUNDATION

Supporting children, adults and families
for better mental health. #letsdostuff

For more information and support for family and friends around
mental health issues, please visit The Shaw Mind Foundation
website at **www.shawmindfoundation.org**

SECTION 7

MEDICATION

Adam: In this section we will approach the subject of medication that can sometimes be prescribed for OCD, anxiety, panic attacks and depression, in parallel to following the PTT approach outlined in this book.

Medication can be a contentious topic for mental health issues, drawing opinion from the whole spectrum of society. The ethos of our PTT approach is about providing sound advice and options for the sufferer and acknowledging that medication is currently one of those options. Beginning a course of prescription medication has to be the choice of the sufferer and must be discussed in detail with a medical specialist. Our PTT approach does not promote prescription medication for OCD, anxiety, panic attacks and related depression, nor does it disapprove of prescription medication if the sufferer feels it is appropriate for their circumstances.

The PTT approach can be used with or without medication, but in keeping with our ethos we feel the detail provided by Lauren below is appropriate, in order for the sufferer to have clarity on options and choice. PTT does, however, believe that while medication, when used correctly and in line with the Medical specialist recommendations, may assist in your recovery, a satisfactory recovery can only be made by using a cognitive-behavioural and compassion-focused approach such as PTT as well.

In my personal story in the first section of this book, I mentioned that I was initially on Fluoxetine (also known as Prozac), the prescription for which began after my major anxiety episode. I also started and stayed with Fluoxetine right through my initial sessions with Lauren and found it to be useful, in that in my critical days it stabilised my mood and put me in a place where I was receptive to the challenges of Lauren's treatment approach. So medication played its part for me at the beginning of my recovery, but (and it is a very big 'but') that's not to say it is for everybody. In fact, we say that it is absolutely possible to undergo the PTT approach WITHOUT needing medication, if you feel you are able. I considered I needed medication because I'd had so many years of troublesome OCD and extreme anxiety, and was at the point of giving up on my life. I seemed to have no space left in my mind to even consider an approach that would need me to do some extra thinking, as I was physically and mentally drained from my illness as well as being very depressed; I could not even bring myself to speak. You may not feel the same as I did; every individual is different, and everyone's level of anxiety and mental health issues is different. This is why the PTT approach encourages the sufferer to decide what is best for him or her when it comes to medication.

 Lauren: Medication can be very helpful for some people and give them the support and boost they need to undertake a therapeutic treatment approach. Not everyone needs medication to follow an approach such as PTT but some people may prefer it. In my clinical experience I have seen many people on medication, and I've noticed how it allows them to engage in treatment and helps stabilise their mood in order to get the best out of treatment. In addition, I have seen many people get better without taking medication.

Current advice states that if you have mild to moderate OCD or anxiety, you do not necessarily need medication to get better. A good course of psychological treatment based on CBT is an effective treatment on its own. However, some people with mild to moderate OCD or anxiety have co-morbid depression and might require medication for their mood, or they might still prefer to take medication to help them in their OCD and anxiety treatment.

If you have a more severe anxiety or obsessional problem, the evidence is that medication can help you alongside a good course of treatment. Again, not everyone in this category needs to take medication; even people with more severe OCD and anxiety can get better without it, but research shows it can help.

The medication that is first considered for OCD and anxiety belongs in a family called Selective Serotonin Reuptake Inhibitors (SSRI). It is a family of anti-depressants that have been proven to be effective for anxiety, OCD and depression. Another group of anti-depressants called Serotonin Norepinephrine Reuptake Inhibitors (SNRI) also have clinical effectiveness and might be prescribed. In some cases, another antidepressant called a tricyclic antidepressant might be prescribed for OCD. Which medication is prescribed will depend on individual factors such as medication history and medical background, and the prescribed doses will vary within a recommended range. Sometimes doctors may even combine medications (called augmentation) for people if it is clinically indicated. These antidepressant medications are not addictive and there is good evidence that they help with OCD, anxiety and depression.

Other medications that can be used for symptom management of anxiety problems, i.e. the physical symptoms of anxiety, are known as beta blockers. These medications are not addictive and can be used in specific situations under the clear advice of a doctor. One medication that can be prescribed for people with Generalised Anxiety Disorder (GAD) is known as Pregabalin. Although this was originally a painkiller for neuropathic difficulties, there is good evidence for its use in GAD. Benzodiazepines are anti-anxiety medications that can be prescribed in emergency situations to provide immediate relief. However, we wouldn't recommend benzodiazepines for long-term management of an anxiety problem because they are addictive and can continue to mask physiological symptoms, enabling those taking such medication to believe they don't need psychological treatment. This can become a safety behaviour and as we now know, this is not helpful. It is highly unlikely that you would be prescribed any of the above drugs without advice that you also undertake a course of psychological treatment.[25]

Some people find that medication works for them alongside a treatment approach. Others aren't keen on medication and can get better following a course of evidenced based psychological treatment.

25 NICE (2005). Obsessive-compulsive disorder and body dysmorphic disorder: treatment. Retrieved from www.nice.org.uk/guidance/cg31.

We suggest that you always talk to your medical practitioner about the options and to understand any side effects of medication.

Just because there are side effects doesn't mean you will get them all, and every person responds differently to them. Even if one particular drug doesn't work for you, another might, so don't worry if you haven't responded to the first medication you have tried.

Medication itself can become a safety behaviour or the cause of obsession and worry about problems, in that some people think that being prescribed medication means they are 'mad', and this is certainly not the case. Or some people think they only got better solely because of the medication, which is of course not true if they have undertaken the hard work in a robust psychological treatment like the PTT approach. Other people might think they are 'weak' if they are prescribed medication and cannot get over the OCD or anxiety on their own. Again, this is not true – we wouldn't tell someone with a physical illness to stop taking medication! So it is not different from taking medication to help with depression and anxiety – both of which have biological roots too, just like physical illnesses.

Equally, some people search the internet to find the perfect medication to overcome their anxiety and OCD but there really is no 'magic pill' for this. Medication might help alleviate some of the symptoms but it won't eliminate them and you will still need a course of good psychological treatment with an approach such as PTT. It is highly unlikely that medication alone will solve your problems and be warned: the quest for the perfect medication can become an obsession itself.

In short, review the options for medication, learn about side effects, speak to your medical practitioner or clinician and decide whether medication is right for you. Our ethos is not to push for or against medication, as we recognise that people can get better with or without it as long as they undertake good psychological treatment such as PTT. For more information on medication, please visit www.shawmindfoundation.org.

SECTION 8

LIFE AFTER ANXIETY:
RECOVERY AND THE PLACE BEYOND

Adam: Aside from successfully launching our global charity, The Shaw Mind Foundation, and producing this recovery approach with Lauren over the last few years, what happened to me post-recovery? Did I just get better and carry on as before? Or did the whole experience change my life forever? Well, if you've read this far, I think you might know the answer already!

So many years of trauma and a recovery that I look upon as almost miraculous – albeit using such simple techniques – meant that my life could never be the same again. Having a wife and five children, I couldn't just fly off around the world in search of some spiritual truth, even if I'd wanted to. Whatever changes needed to happen had to be made much closer to home and had to involve my family. My illness had put them through hell and I owed them big time for all the occasions that I couldn't be with them, either through work or because I was mentally incapable of a proper relationship with them.

Today, I consider myself a much more empathetic and compassionate person than I have ever been. My relationship with my children now is wonderful. I don't claim to be the perfect parent – only a fool would – but now I am able to give them the time, love and support they need without the distractions of anxiety and OCD swirling around my head. As a family, we are honest with each other. The kids know that daddy has 'quirks', and they don't see these as odd or strange because we've talked about them openly and honestly – and therefore we've normalised them. We think it's vital that mental health issues are discussed, and we've talked about my difficulties using the scale of severity that Lauren introduced in Chapter 3 of the first part of this book. They know that most of the time I'm on the 'fine' end of the scale and just very occasionally I'm a little bit on the other side. That's OK with them; they understand and accept what is going on because they see it as part of me.

I'm also far less quick to judge and condemn than I used to be. In the past, so many of my responses were knee-jerk ones. Today, I think carefully before I respond, even if someone really upsets me, and I also put myself in the shoes of the person I'm responding to. What's going on for them? What factors are present in their lives which makes them operate the way they do? I see now that when I was anxious and unhappy, I found it easy to transfer those negative feelings to other people; snapping at them, putting them down and being a dictator at work. Through the PTT treatment approach I've understood how being at ease with yourself reduces your anxieties and prevents you from offloading your pain on others. For me, empathy and compassion are learned behaviours and while I still have the 'tiger' inside me to drive things forward and make them happen, I have learned how to harness this drive for positive outcomes that does not involve steamrollering others in order to get what I want. Ten years ago I was very critical of people because I wasn't happy and didn't like myself much. Today, that situation has completely changed.

As you'll recall, when I was poorly I made a promise to myself that I would make my wife and children proud, and if I recovered I would devote time, money and energy into helping others in my situation. As I started to get better I found myself thinking about this promise and how I could make it a reality. Because there are obvious difficulties worldwide for OCD and anxiety sufferers in getting sound access to treatment, it struck me that a self-help approach was an obvious solution – and so here we are!

Our prime aim at this point can be found in our mission statement (at the front of the book), which is to focus on our own charity foundation and those charities around us that specifically help those suffering through any mental illness.

I am lucky in that I'm able to devote the resources to this and ensure it has a global presence to reach all those in need, though I had to ask myself, 'Do I also have the time?' At the point I came up with the strategy of building Lauren's expertise into a recovery approach and ensuring it was accessible for all, the answer was 'no'. I still owned and ran a large legal services business which demanded so much of that precious time.

As it happened, an offer from a well-known corporate entity based in the UK to buy my legal services business came in just at the time I was mulling over my plans. In the past I'd have been very resistant to the idea of a sale; I'd built up this business from a spare bedroom, so why should I let it go? Now, however, I had two good reasons – I'd be able to spend more time with my family now I was recovered and in the best mental health of my life, and I'd also have the flexibility to pursue my strategy about helping others with mental health issues through The Shaw Mind Foundation (www.shawmindfoundation.org) as well as reaching out to fellow sufferers with this recovery approach.

After accepting the offer, we decided as a family to make a conscious decision to temporarily relocate to the island of Lanzarote in the Canaries, which had been the scene of some of my most acute periods of anxiety; I really wanted to go back there, face the demons of the past and finally lay them to rest, which is exactly what happened.

However, the idea of having more time didn't quite work out the way I envisaged, as I still sit on the board of directors of the company I built and sold, and I also have other business interests outside legal services. I am driven by business and ventures that make differences and improvements to the community as a whole, so I'm still busy in that sense, although I am able to spend more quality time with my family than before now that I am not shouldering the burden of owning and running a large company. That said, I seemed to spend a lot less time in Lanzarote over this temporary period of relocation than I'd hoped, as I was more often than not working back in the UK due to my appetite and enthusiasm for business.

I understand that most survivors of OCD and anxiety aren't all fortunate enough to find themselves in my personal and professional position post-recovery. Many sufferers may have little choice other than to go back to their occupations and pick up where they left off. But that doesn't mean the future cannot be embraced and lived to a new set of values. I don't have the perfect life – nobody does – but

I now see that life is a journey, not a fight. I accept and embrace this journey because, in common with anyone who has recovered from an illness, physical or mental, I feel life is a blessing. Whatever it throws at me – good or bad – I accept as part of that journey.

The PTT recovery approach evolved from the techniques which Lauren introduced to me, but is also derived from our combined experience, wisdom and expertise which eventually evolved into the PTT approach we have shared with you. It taught me that accepting and embracing aren't just ways of controlling anxiety. In fact, they apply to your whole life. You can fight life, wearing the resulting scars and carrying around the trauma of battle, or you can choose to accept what is, change those parts you can change and let go of the rest. This way, you will find peace in your life, and peace is much better than war.

People in battles will always have a high state of anxiety, are constantly alert for danger and can make very rash decisions. Fighting simply preserves and encourages all the symptoms that fuel unnecessary anxiety. While we know that certain amounts of anxiety are essential in life, over-indulging anxiety by letting your thoughts and fears control you to a point where it causes great distress offers absolutely no benefit to brain or body. Alternatively, if you choose to live your life by using the PTT process of accepting and embracing any situation in life, good or bad, then I assure you that you will make better judgements, better decisions and more rational responses to potential conflict with others. Always remember that letting go and not being in control of your thoughts, and simply letting them be there and accepted for what they are, in fact gives you complete control of your mind and your mental well-being. Just as importantly, it gives you control to focus on your aspirations for life.

People often say that they deal with whatever life throws at them, and while that's OK for those people, it's not how I choose to live my life now. I do the opposite – I throw myself at life and let it deal with me. I don't spend too much time pondering over things, and I certainly don't try to figure out the whys and wherefores of my illness. I accept that it happened to me and I embrace it as part of who I am. In short, I live in and for the moment and I try to say 'yes' to new ideas and other people's points of view as much as I can, because that way I learn something about other people and I challenge myself too.

I was always prepared to take a risk in life, but now I see the practical benefits of this, and once you're free of anxiety you're also free to make the choices and take the risks you may previously have considered a person like you to be incapable of. Being free of anxiety enables you to do those things in life you've always wanted to do, to take a chance and see where you go. It's not always easy, but I try to see what I've been through as positively as possible, and I think it's vital to take something positive out of every situation. If it hasn't gone your way this time, so what? You'll have learned something for next time and you'll keep trying until you achieve what you set out to do. I believe in aspiring to something, working hard for something you'd like in life. Aspiration makes us grow and it's good for both physical and mental well-being. No athlete ever got to the Olympics expecting to come last, and even if that happens, he or she can tell themselves that very, very few ever get to where they've got to.

That said, if it all goes wrong, don't be too hard on yourself. As ever and as stipulated in our PTT approach, simply accept what is. If you can change the situation, great; if you can't, then embrace what you have and learn to appreciate it for what it is. And wherever possible, don't criticise other people. We all roughly have the same amount of faults as each other, so don't waste your time and effort criticising other people's faults. Instead, focus on your own development and do it with love and compassion for yourself and others.

For many years, my anxiety led me to be my harshest critic, whether this be through my illness or when something didn't go quite right in my business world. In short, I made the mistake of trying to be Superman. I would expect perfection from myself every day in my professional life. I would have a massive 'to do' list to complete before the end of the day. And if I dropped any of the balls I was juggling, I would really come down on myself. It was only after recovering through the PTT approach that I suddenly realised and asked the questions 'Why was I giving myself a hard time? Would I ever use such harsh words when talking to any of my children, family, friends, colleagues or clients?' Of course I wouldn't; I'd be caring and nurturing and look for ways to support and encourage their confidence rather than knock them down. Therefore, I now live my life **ACCEPTING** my faults and being kinder to myself. This doesn't mean that I'm less focused, ambitious or professional. Far from it – in fact, this helps me to focus on the things that I love to do and that I am good at. By **EMBRACING** kindness to myself I have also stopped feeling guilty when I want to do something for myself. The time I now take out for me can only be good for my loved ones, family and friends as they get to see a much more stress-free Adam who is open to opportunities.

> *Kindness in words creates confidence. Kindness in thinking creates profoundness. Kindness in giving creates love.*　　**Lao Tzu**

Finally, let me leave you with this personal thought which is relevant to the ethos of our PTT recovery approach and one that I try to live by every day post-recovery. It works for me, and I hope it will work for you too.

> *If you don't take chances ... then expect no change; expect an average life at best. If you do take chances, then expect the unexpected and with the unexpected, anything can happen and that's more fun; that's living a life and not just simply existing.*

CONCLUSION

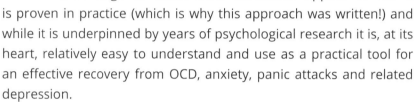

Lauren and Adam: The PTT approach – so named because it encourages sufferers of anxiety and obsessional problems from mild to severe levels to go towards the root of their fears – is based on sound clinical principles and is aimed at all sufferers, no matter how large or small their difficulties appear to be. It is proven in practice (which is why this approach was written!) and while it is underpinned by years of psychological research it is, at its heart, relatively easy to understand and use as a practical tool for an effective recovery from OCD, anxiety, panic attacks and related depression.

Many congratulations! We're now at the end of _Pulling the Trigger_ and we both hope that the personal and practical journey we've taken you on has been useful, rewarding and life-changing. We know how difficult it is to embark on this journey; how challenging it can be to embrace everything we've talked about and apply it to your own situation. And we also know that to do this successfully can bring untold rewards in terms of a life free from OCD, anxiety, panic attacks and related depression.

The latter is a vitally important point. By following the PTT approach, not only do you get your life back, but you discover whole new avenues of experience available to you, that you may have not previously considered. Taking control of OCD, anxiety, panic attacks and related depression and freeing yourself from its power is extremely liberating, so be prepared to discover a new you that is ready to open doors, take advantage of opportunities and explore new ways of living. Our PTT approach and its principles are not just about survival and recovery, but can help harness and shape your future for the place beyond recovery.

And why stop at recovery? We can make our mental health issues the biggest positive influence in our life. They've given us the platform we need to take action and create a fulfilled life for the future. Our mental health issues have created and given us a strength we did not know we had; a resilient strength. Think about it, you have a 100 per cent success rate even before you started this recovery approach; you have survived every day no matter how bad the distress or torment has been. Use this view of your strength to drive your courage forward in embracing the PTT approach. The mental health issues we suffer from actually have a huge positive impact if we approach them correctly. They have helped us lay the foundations in learning and understanding our minds and behaviour more than we ever knew. Don't be afraid of this fact: accept it, embrace it and thank it for allowing you to learn from it and therefore educate yourself on the way to living a more fulfilled life with positivity, confidence, but just as importantly, complete control of your mental health well-being. Life is there for the taking; go to it and embrace every moment of it.

If you've followed the PTT approach carefully, you will know that at its heart are the concepts of **Accept**, **Embrace** and **Control**. We outlined these concepts very carefully and we appreciate that, at first, there is a lot to take in. The good news is, however, that once you have an understanding of PTT and are able to implement it into your recovery – and you are able to see the thoughts for what they are – you will be able to use the PTT approach as soon as you notice anxiety creeping up. In time, this will naturally reduce intrusive thoughts and urges as they will simply not ignite your anxiety radar any more.

Now let's recap some of the main points in this book, so you can easily refer to them as you go through your recovery process and beyond. The 'beyond' bit is particularly important, as there are many lessons contained in these pages that point the way to a life that can be led with more happiness and success. Think of the book as a manual not only for survival and recovery, but as a handbook for leading a more fulfilled life generally by using the relatively simple but highly effective PTT approach.

Anxiety and obsessional problems come in all shapes and sizes. But at their core, all the problems we have addressed in this book can be broken down into their components – triggers, thoughts, emotions, physiological symptoms and behavioural responses. The trigger is the event, which can be anything, including a place, thought, sensation, urge, experience etc. which starts off the unhelpful cycle. The thought is how we then interpret the trigger which will take the form of a number of thinking problems, usually a catastrophic interpretation of events which are now considered a 'threat'. How we feel about this is our emotional response, normally anxiety but can also be depression and other emotions. Our bodies usually go into fight, flight or freeze mode at this point, and we experience a number of uncomfortable physiological symptoms. Our behavioural responses are how we then respond to these threats and emotional and physiological sensations, and usually involve avoidance, seeking reassurance, mental rumination and creative safety behaviours.

Anxiety itself is a primal response to threat, better known as 'fight, flight or freeze'. It's a defence mechanism and we all need a little anxiety in our lives to keep us functioning actively. However, anxiety becomes debilitating and dangerous when we attach importance to it that inflates its position in our lives. This includes panic attacks – a heightened manifestation of anxiety symptoms. Attempting to control thoughts, push them aside, invent safety behaviours to suppress them or avoid anxiety, and avoiding situations in which the thoughts and feelings of anxiety may occur, actually make problems with OCD and anxiety much worse.

We know that OCD is an obsessional disorder sitting on a background of anxiety in which sufferers attach meanings to unwanted thoughts, then employ a range of mental and physical behavioural strategies in an attempt to rid themselves of the thoughts and the anxious feelings. If, for example, you know the only way of getting rid of the thought and to feel less anxious is by counting in multiples of seven, or repeating a certain phrase to yourself, or replacing the thought with a 'neutral' or 'safe' thought, then the logical next step is to do that thing. The intrusive thought goes away and you're safe – until the next time it pops into your head and causes you distress. That is OCD.

The 'meaning' side of OCD has three parts; the first is the **Catastrophic interpretation** ('What's the worst that could happen?'), followed by the **Magnified Duty** interpretation ('I've had this terrible thought and it's my fault if something happens'). The last part is the **Perceived Control** aspect ('I've had this thought, but there is something I can do to control it, or make it go away').

OCD can and does attach itself to anything, and while its causes are varied, the fact that you are a sufferer is not your fault. We all have unwelcome thoughts. It's how we choose to interpret them and then how we respond to that interpretation which determines how much of a problem they will become for us.

We call responses to such thoughts **compulsions**, **rituals** or **safety behaviours**. People with OCD and/or anxiety seek comfort in compulsions and safety behaviours because they see them as safety valves for their worries. They can be both physical and mental. We call these '**safety behaviours**' because they are actions that anxiety sufferers carry out to feel safe from their worries. This might bring relief at first, but the anxiety will not be sated, and will continuously require more rituals, compulsions and safety behaviours. These rituals, compulsions and safety behaviours reinforce the strength of the catastrophic meaning, bringing increasing anxiety and disturbance to everyday life. These behaviours actually reinforce the message of danger.

As we've mentioned, our **PTT** approach has, at its core, three principal concepts: Accept, Embrace and Control.

- **Accepting** that you have an anxiety problem or obsessional problem is key, as is accepting that this is your current state of mind. And within this, accepting that you're having unwanted or uncomfortable thoughts and uncomfortable feelings (both emotional and physiological) is the first step towards recovery. This stops the fight and although this is still uncomfortable for you, it feeds the anxiety, OCD and panic attacks no further: you have culled the growth. (Refer to Adam's conclusion page 127).

- **Embracing** those thoughts involves going towards them and welcoming them in, no matter how fearful you might feel. Initially, this is hard work and requires courage. Remember – don't get 'fight' mixed up with 'courage'. You are not offering this illness a fight; you are having the courage to call its bluff and see it for what it is – a fake! Embracing means doing what the anxiety is telling you not to do or avoid. Embracing will get easier over time. Soon enough the process will feel more natural and you will habituate to the feared situation, and this will become less and less scary. (Refer to Adam's conclusion page 177).

- **Controlling** those thoughts and fears occurs, ironically, by not 'controlling' them in the conventional sense of suppressing them and trying to rid yourself of the thoughts, urges and anxiety sensations, but by allowing them in, noticing them, but not judging them. As a consequence you also take further control in this sense of you now deciding when you are going to interact with them and not the other way around, where they try to control and dictate to you. Control is also understanding and accepting that it's OK not to be in control of your thoughts, urges and sensations. (Refer to Adam's conclusion page 192).

Once you have begun your journey to 'Pulling the Trigger', you may start asking yourself 'Is that it? Is that all there is to this – **Accept**, **Embrace**, **Control**?' The process really is that simple; what may make it seem so complex at times is understanding that it's OK to allow the doubt to be there through your survival and recovery journey. In fact, it's critical to your recovery. You need the doubt, anxiety, panic and OCD in all its glory to start the process of **Accept** and **Embrace** which begins the desensitising process. Do not question the simplicity of it; embrace it by facing the fear you have associated with it and have the courage to see it through correctly. Don't fall into the trap of worrying why it is so simple. The way to deal with OCD and anxiety is to do the exact opposite to what your mind initially perceives as the natural thing to do, e.g. run away from it, fear it, try and get rid of the thoughts, go over and over it in your head to try and rationalise with it and figure it out, and worse still, continue to question it. If you are feeling the anxiety and wanting to question it (which is a guarantee) then you are indeed going through the correct process in 'Pulling the Trigger'.

The aim of recovering from anxiety-based mental illness is not to rid yourself of the thoughts, urges or feelings you get from the illness, but the very opposite in allowing yourself to be exposed to them and embracing them. **Try and look at it like recovering from a broken arm, or a torn muscle or even a cut. Can you heal your broken arm, muscle or cut by analysing it, worrying about it, fighting it or by willing yourself for it to be better? Of course not, you have to accept it first, and then engage in an evidenced based treatment approach in order to heal. The exact same principle applies to anxiety.** Have courage and take the journey – you will never look back.

And finally, it is very important to treat ourselves with compassion and care throughout our struggle with mental health problems and during our recovery. This is very difficult to do, especially if it feels that things are not improving despite your best efforts. It is easy to get caught up in self-criticism and self-blame. But remember, despite being overwhelmed, you are not to blame for these problems, and you are a worthwhile person and deserve to get better. We all need care to get better and care takes many forms. One of the most important forms is self–care; being kind and compassionate to ourselves. This does not mean avoid the hard parts of the treatment programme, in fact quite the opposite! Engaging in challenging our anxieties and OCD, and facing up to them IS treating ourselves with compassion as we are telling ourselves we can, will, and most importantly deserve to get better.

For further information on our PTT approach and other self help and support books for mental health recovery, see www.pulling-the-trigger.com.

Also available is The Pulling the Trigger Juniors and Teenagers Edition approach, including guidance for parents. This definitive recovery approach for OCD, anxiety, panic attacks and related depression is specifically designed and aimed at helping young people and their families on their path to recovery. This book is specifically tailored for a younger readership, plus their parents.

Adam: Anxiety-based mental illness robbed me of my years through childhood to early adolescence. It's a devastating, debilitating, and above all, very lonely illness which sucks the life out of you and constantly questions your sanity. During childhood such emotions cause confusion and internal turmoil, so much so that even at an early age you question whether life is worth living. This simply cannot be allowed to happen to our children and teenagers. We won't allow it to happen, and with the passion which is driven by our mission statement, we will help children and teenagers survive and indeed recover from anxiety-based mental illness. We will support and show parents and family members of sufferers how to spot the signs of this illness and what can be done to help loved ones recover, embrace their life and live it to their potential. The Juniors and Teenagers edition, including guidance for parents, makes me so very proud as it gives me the chance to go back in time to over thirty years ago and write to my then self as a lost child, debilitated by anxiety-based mental illness. It also gives me the chance to have an edition of 'Pulling the Trigger' in which I can have my own children and their future children in mind and show them the correct way on how to survive, recover and beat this illness and live a positive and enriched life.

www.pulling-the-trigger.com/recovery-support-books

 Lauren and Adam: We sincerely hope you have enjoyed and embraced the journey we've shared with you in this book and the approach contained within it, and that some or all of it has given you the tools and the inspiration you need to embark on your own journey out of the grip of OCD, anxiety, panic attacks and related depression. We hope that your journey is a fruitful one, and that it leads to a life of peace, contentment and fulfillment. Survival and recovery is possible and can be inevitable, we promise (please visit www.pulling-the-trigger.com).

BIBLIOGRAPHY

American Psychiatric Association. (2013). *Diagnostic and Statistical Manual of Mental Disorders* (5th ed.). Washington, DC: American Psychiatric Association.

Beck, A. T. & Emery, G., with Greenberg, R. L. (1985). *Anxiety Disorders and Phobias: A Cognitive Perspective.* New York: Basic Books.

Beck, J. S. (2011). *Cognitive Behavior Therapy: Basics and Beyond* (2nd ed). New York: Guilford.

Clark, D. M. (1986). A cognitive approach to panic. *Behaviour Research and Therapy*, 24(4), 461–70.

Clark, D. M. (1989) Anxiety states: Panic and generalized anxiety. In **Hawton**, Keith (Ed); **Salkovskis, Paul M. (Ed); Kirk, Joan (Ed); Clark, David M. (Ed),** (1989). *Cognitive Behaviour Therapy for Psychiatric Problems: A Practical Guide. Oxford Medical Publications* (pp. 52–96). New York, NY, US: Oxford University Press.

Dimidjian, S., Hollon, S. D., Dobson, K. S., Schmaling, K. B., Kohlenberg, R. J., Addis, M. E. & Atkins, D. C. (2006). Randomized trial of behavioral activation, cognitive therapy, and antidepressant medication in the acute treatment of adults with major depression. *Journal of Consulting and Clinical Psychology*, 74(4), 658.

Dugas, M. J. & Robichaud M. (2006) *Categories of Worry Strategy Adopted from Cognitive-Behavioral Treatment for Generalized Anxiety Disorder: From Science to Practice.* New York: Routledge.

Gilbert, P. (2010). *The Compassionate Mind: A New Approach to Life's Challenge.* Oakland, CA: New Harbinger Publications.

Merton, R. K. (1948). The self-fulfilling prophecy. *Antioch Review*, 8, 193–210.

NICE. (2005). Obsessive-compulsive disorder and body dysmorphic disorder: treatment. Retrieved from www.nice.org.uk/guidance/cg31.

Rachman, S. (1997). A cognitive theory of obsessions. *Behaviour Research and Therapy*, 35, 793–802.

Salkovskis, P. M. (1985). Obsessive-compulsive problems: A cognitive behavioural analysis. *Behaviour Research and Therapy*, 11, 271–7.

Salkovskis, P. M. (1999). Understanding and treating obsessive-compulsive disorder. *Behaviour Research and Therapy*, 37, S29–S52.

Salkovskis, P. M., Wroe A. L., Gledhill A., Morrison N., Forrester E., Richards C., Reynolds M. & Thorpe S. (2000). Responsibility attitudes and interpretations are characteristic of obsessive compulsive disorder. *Behaviour Research and Therapy*, 38(4), 347–72.

Shafran, R., Thordarson, D. S. & Rachman, S. (1996). Thought-action fusion in obsessive compulsive disorder. *Journal of Anxiety Disorders,* 10(5), 379–91.

Van Oppen, P. & Arntz, A. (1994). Cognitive therapy for obsessive compulsive disorder. *Behaviour Research and Therapy,* 32(1), 79–87.

WHO – The World Health Organisation www.who.int/en/.

INDEX

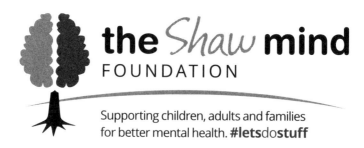

Supporting children, adults and families
for better mental health. **#lets**do**stuff**

Sign up to our charity, The Shaw Mind Foundation

www.shawmindfoundation.org

and keep in touch with us; we would love to hear from you.

*We aim to bring to an end the suffering and despair caused
by mental health issues. Our goal is to make help and support
available for every single person in society, from all walks of life.
We will never stop offering hope. These are our promises.*

Additonal copies of the tables from this book can be downloaded from the **Pulling**the**trigger**® website.

Please visit the link below:

www.pulling-the-trigger.com/resources